The Yoga of Spiritual Devotion

The Yoga of Spiritual Devotion

A Modern Translation of the Narada Bhakti Sutras

Prem Prakash

Inner Traditions International
Rochester, Vermont

Inner Traditions International
One Park Street
Rochester, Vermont 05767
www.gotoit.com

Library of Congress Cataloging-in-Publication Data
Prem Prakash, 1959–
The yoga of spiritual devotion : a modern translation of the Narada bhakti sutras / Prem Prakash.
p. cm.
ISBN 0-89281-664-3 (pbk. : alk. paper)
1. Nārada. Bhaktisūtra. 2. Bhakti.
3. Yoga, Bhakti. I. Title.
BL1214.32.B53P74 1998 97-49646
294.5'43—dc21 CIP

Printed and bound in Canada

10 9 8 7 6 5 4 3 2 1

Text design and layout by Kristin Camp
This book was typeset in Sabon

Distributed to the book trade in Canada by Publishers Group West (PGW), Toronto
Distributed to the book trade in the United Kingdom by Deep Books, London
Distributed to the book trade in Australia by Gemcraft Books, Burwood
Distributed to the book trade in New Zealand by Tandem Press, Auckland
Distributed to the book trade in South Africa by Alternative Books, Ferndale

Contents

I dedicate this book to you, dear reader, with a prayer that it will help bring you nearer to peace and joy. Along the path I have stepped on many thorns. I hope this leaves fewer to pierce your beautiful feet.

Acknowledgments

I would like to thank the following people for their assistance in the preparation of this book: Baba Hari Dass, my yoga guru, for supporting and providing direction for this project; Georg Feuerstein, who has done so much for the transmission of yoga to the West, for carefully reviewing the manuscript and offering valuable suggestions; Suneel Beyers for his help with sources and enthusiastically preparing the devanagari script and word index; and Lesley Ambika Gibbs for her helpful advice and patient assistance with the preparation of the manuscript. I'd also like to thank the fine people at Inner Traditions International, who are a delight to work with, notably Jon Graham, David Raizman, Rowan Jacobsen, Mary Elder Jacobsen, Serena Fox, and my very skilled editor, Susan Davidson.

Author's Preface

Here is a doctrine at which you will laugh.
It may be important to great thinkers to
examine the world; to explain and despise
it. But I think it is only important to
love the world, not to despise it, not for
us to hate each other, but to be able to
regard the world and ourselves and all
*beings with love, admiration and respect.**

Siddhartha, by Herman Hesse

The bhakti sutras of Narada form the principal text of the yoga of spiritual devotion. As Patanjali's sutras are to the raja yoga schools and the Upanishads to the Vedanta schools, likewise is the significance of the Narada sutras to bhakti

---

*Herman Hesse, *Siddhartha,* trans. Hilda Rosner (New York: New Directions, 1951), 148–49.

yoga. For those unfamiliar with the form, many traditional yogic teachings are presented in a series of terse verses whose meaning binds them together into a *sutra,* literally "thread," as in a thread on which is strung a garland of fragrant flowers. A teacher may then write an original commentary on the verses for the purpose of helping the flowers blossom in a reader's consciousness.

There are several translations of the Narada Bhakti Sutras in English, but I am not aware of a translation and commentary completed by a Westerner. The existing commentaries all share one shortcoming—they fail to address the nature of bhakti in a manner that does justice to the psychological needs of twentieth- (and soon to be twenty-first-) century Westerners and other global citizens. The traditional Indian approach to bhakti is oriented toward students from a nontechnological society with cultural and religious premises that are at great variance with those of contemporary Western society. The ancient Indian teachers of bhakti yoga never had to contend with many of the social and personal issues that face present-day students, issues such as the value of personal freedom, the more egalitarian status of women, and the widespread Judeo-Christian guilt over some ancient concept of a pre-birth "original sin."

Even with yoga having spread from its birthplace in India and taken firm root in the West, there are still few significant works on the bhakti tradition available to sincere students. This is of concern because the teachings of bhakti, I believe, will exercise a great influence over the future development of yoga in the modern world. Yoga in the West is taking a form contrary to the world-negating view that has developed in India, and this may prove to be the West's gift to the yogic tradition. The yoga of the next millenium will, in my opinion, provide aspirants with philosophies and practices that will enable them to be both citizens and yogis, to be in the world but not of it. This is where bhakti, with its positive approach toward love, relationships, and activities in the world, will be most significant.

In his *Yoga: The Technology of Ecstasy,* Georg Feuerstein remarks on the current status of resources available for Westerners and alludes to the potential for bhakti to exert a strong influence on the future of yoga. He writes, "The history of the bhakti cult and subsequent movement is vastly complex, and modern scholarship has only scratched the surface. What is clear, however, is that India has not only had its share of world-denying mystics but can also take pride in many generations of thousands of love-intoxicated seekers and realizers."* Yoga in contemporary Western culture is not cultivating world-denying mystics, but with the proper resources and training in bhakti, the West can produce love-intoxicated seekers and realizers. It is my hope that this book will serve as one of those resources.

In addition to my hope that this book will be of value for Westerners, I also present it as an offering to our Eastern elders, those who have kept the lamp of yoga burning for so many millenia. In light of our burgeoning global village, I hope this book may serve as a bridge between the traditions of Indian yoga and the birth of Western yoga. Though Narada pours the old wine, we in the West must drink from bottles of our own making. Our goal should not be to become like our Indian predecessors, but to cultivate our own vineyards and produce our own vintages.

As for myself, I am American by birth and have been a

---

*Georg Feuerstein, *Yoga: The Technology of Ecstasy* (Los Angeles: Jeremy Tarcher, 1989), 52.

practicing yogi since 1979, having studied formally with several teachers from different lineages. I was hardly born enlightened on a lotus flower. My spiritual progress is primarily the result of stubbornness and grace; I am a fool who came into some wisdom by persisting with my folly and trying to be receptive to my teachers. If I can progress on the spiritual path, so can anyone who reads this book and commits to love.

I received initiation into my yogic name from the silent yogi Baba Hari Dass. In 1990, Baba Hari Dass gave me permission to teach. Since 1991 I have served as director of the Green Mountain School of Yoga, where I continue to teach traditional ashtanga yoga.

A Note on the Translation

This book is intended to serve two purposes, which, while mutually supportive, result in two different styles of presentation of the romanized renderings of Sanskrit terms. One purpose is to satisfy those students who wish to study the sutras in their original Sanskrit. This is addressed in the translation and word analysis of the sutras, which are meant to be accurate reflections of the language that Narada used to present his message. The English transliterations from the Sanskrit are given with the necessary diacritical marks in order to meet the requirements of formal scholarly and scriptural study.

The other purpose of this book is to assist those who wish to cultivate spiritual devotion as a means to enlightenment. This is the basis for the commentary, which is intended to be accessible to aspirants at all levels of familiarity with Sanskrit. In my commentary, English renderings from the Sanskrit are presented phonetically in order to help bring alive the beauty and poetry of Sanskrit, without the diacritical marks which often prove visually distracting to the nonspecialist.

Introduction

Yoga is the science and art of the union of the individual soul with God. This union is not something to be generated or attained, per se; it already exists, needing only to be realized and expressed to its fullest potential. In the same manner that waves are already part of the ocean, being the very power of the ocean, likewise are the individual souls to God. The goal of *bhakti yoga,* the path of spiritual devotion, is the realization of this relationship between the soul and God.

In the yogic traditions God's nature is described as *sat-chit-ananda:* eternal life, infinite consciousness, and limitless bliss. God is the One—the timeless, universal consciousness of unconditional love, as well as the source of the souls and their own creative impetus. The individual soul is a spark from the sun of God that experiences the universe during a journey in the manifest worlds.

The individual soul is the same sat-chit-ananda nature as God, but the soul's voyage in the spheres of relative existence engenders a confusion of identity. Through identification with the various bodies she produces, which are the vehicles that make the voyage possible, the soul forgets her true nature. She comes to believe she *is* those bodies, and hence, that she is mortal, limited, and subject to suffering. This confusion is not due to any original sin deserving punishment from God; it is a primal energy that is itself the seed of the cosmic drama of separation and reunion.

Suffering reaches its most poignant state in a human being, awakening a sense that "all is not well." This recognition of elementary dissatisfaction is the beginning of the conscious spiritual pilgrimage by the soul. She begins to search for answers that address the causes of suffering and its appeasement. The contemplative power of the soul, the intuition, begins to raise the Great Question, the *atma-vichara:* "Who am I?"

The soul spends many incarnations exploring this question and the multitude of answers available in the world. Finally she reaches the point where the atma-vichara becomes the primary influence in life, and the search for a satisfactory answer motivates the undertaking of spiritual practice.

The yogic tradition provides two principal paths of spiritual practice. One is the path of *jnana yoga,* the yoga of wisdom, for those oriented toward answering the atma-vichara in terms of sat (eternal truth). The jnana yogi performs a dissection of the eternal soul from its bodily vehicles and external environment. Through this process the soul realizes herself as distinct from all that is temporal and prone to suffering.

The jnana yogi applies the axiom Neti, neti, "not this, not this," to all phenomena that can be identified as being transient, until what alone is eternal is distilled. Within the context of sat, the temporal forms are realized as insentient manifestations resulting from the intercourse of objects, senses, and mind. The soul is realized as the eternal conscious witness to this process of nature.

The second primary yogic path is that of bhakti yoga, or the yoga of spiritual devotion. It is this path that this book adresses. Bhakti yoga is for those oriented toward answering the atma-vichara in terms of ananda (blissful love). The bhakti yogi performs a dissection of pure love from all that contains a contamination of selfishness. By making love his polestar, the bhakti yogi follows its light along the path of life until the soul realizes it is one with that light.

The bhakti yogi does not undertake processes involving discrimination against phenomena, for to him all phenomena are reflections of God. He seeks to see all form as partial manifestations of *shakti*, God's creative, intelligent energy. Within the context of ananda, the temporal is realized as the reflection of the eternal, and the soul is realized as the expression of God.

A comparison of these two paths is provided in this book (verses 25–33). Also in this text is an examination of the roles played in spiritual development by *karma yoga* (selfless activity) and *raja yoga* (Patanjali's system of meditation). For the moment it will suffice to say that, while all paths lead to the mountain summit, these bhakti sutras declare that spiritual devotion is the simplest, easiest, and most accessible (verses 58–60).

The Narada Bhakti Sutras are considered to have been composed sometime around the twelfth century A.D. It is possible that they were transmitted orally before being circulated in writing. The authorship is attributed to Narada, an archetypal figure of spiritual devotion mentioned throughout millennia of yogic writings.

Narada is said to be a realized sage who travels throughout the universe, often singing and playing the *vina*, a stringed instrument of India. His mission is the dissemination of the teachings of bhakti yoga, and his pastime is participation in ecstatic *kirtan* (chants and songs to God). Some believe that when a kirtan becomes highly charged it will attract Narada, whose subtle presence can be experienced by the participants.

The contentions that Narada is a figure of antiquity and somehow the author of these sutras, a pseudonym employed by the author of these sutras, or some other possibility are all, for practical purposes, equally plausible. The work is neither elevated nor diminished by the status of its author. The Narada Bhakti Sutras are revered because they are a concise summation of an authentic spiritual path and they provide a thorough set of guidelines by which an aspirant can attain Self-realization. Questions of scholarship can remain with scholars. The experience of God awaits those who practice the yoga described in this text.

Verse and Commentary

अथातो भक्तिं व्याख्यास्यामः ।

athāto bhaktiṃ vyākhyāsyāmaḥ

atha—*now, in a spirit of auspiciousness*
ataḥ—*commence*
bhaktiṃ—*bhakti (spiritual devotion)*
vyākhyāsyāmaḥ—*we shall expound*

Verse 1:
Now, in a spirit of auspiciousness, we shall commence to expound on bhakti—spiritual devotion.

Atha, "now," is regularly used in yogic writings as a general introduction to a subject. In addition to its exoteric definition, the word *atha* carries this meaning: Now, in this present moment, should the student give his full attention to this text. The aspirant should hold his mind in a state of focused concentration, of contemplation, of immediacy, in order that the deep truths of these teachings can be assimilated. The bhakti sutras are not intended as casual reading; they are instructions for the attainment of the supreme goal of human life—divine love. The author begins by asking us to be alert, receptive, and appreciative of the treasures that are before us and that, together, will be explored.

As stated in the introduction, bhakti yoga, the path of spiritual devotion, is considered one of the two main yogic paths. Practically, however, all spiritual practice has devotion as its keystone. Without devotion, jnana yoga becomes dry intellectualization, karma yoga dilutes into mere social service, and raja yoga will not bear its fruit because it is undertaken for personal, rather than selfless, reasons. One who practices meditation solely for his own spiritual development may advance on the path but will fail to attain the supreme goal. This failure is because his practice is limited to a desire for his individual accomplishment, reinforcing the egoistic knot of separative consciousness that spiritual practice is intended to untie.

Devotion is actually nothing other than love. To be devoted means to engage with love. The Sanskrit root of *bhakti* is *bhaj,* "to engage with affection." This text will deal with the nature of supreme love—love for God, love for all: how it is cultivated and nourished, and how its fruits are enjoyed.

Contrary to fundamentalist dogma, devotion to the Divine is not a sectarian practice, honoring one idea of God to the exclusion, and even the persecution, of other ideas. All forms are equally applicable for devotion and all bear the same fruit. The experiences of great yogis such as Paramahamsa Ramakrishna bear testimony to this fact. Sri Ramakrishna personally underwent disciplines that resulted in his direct experience of the Divine in the forms of Kali, Hanuman, Jesus, Mohammed, and others.

Our stresses, anxieties, pains, and problems arise because we do not see the world, others, or even ourselves as worthy of love. The development of spiritual devotion does not change anyone or anything; it heals this diseased perception. When the dew is rolled away from our eyes we perceive the worthiness of all beings to be loved, and we take delight in being a channel for the manifestation of love in this world. The world itself is then transformed from an arena of struggle for the mundane personality into a place where a spiritual personality has a purpose and a vocation.

Narada begins by reminding us that we have traveled far enough along the spiritual path that we are entitled to learn these teachings. It is a precious opportunity, not one to be squandered. With a concentrated mind and grateful heart we can respectfully contemplate this scripture and plumb its depths. There are many subtle gems in this mine. Let us be among those who realize its riches.

सा त्वस्मिन् परमप्रेम रुपा ।

sā tvasmin paramaprema rūpā

sā—*that [spiritual devotion]*
tvasmin—*only that*
parama—*supreme*
prema—*love*
rūpā—*nature of*

Verse 2:
The nature of spiritual devotion is the supreme love.

Supreme love is the love of God. The love of God is the only love that exists. All expressions of love are manifestations of this supreme love through limited beings in temporal environments. Even the smallest wave expresses the ocean and can be appreciated as such, but even the largest wave is limited compared to the ocean and should be humble as such.

The love of God is not love *for* God at the exclusion of anything else. For love to be supreme it must avail itself of no limitations. Any limitation on love, by definition, makes it less than supreme.

Devotion, or love, is present in every gesture of kindness, sympathy, and compassion extended by a living being to anything in creation. Materialists begin learning the ways of love by loving what is of the world, eventually coming to a love that is greater than the world. Their brief and less-than-complete experiences of love are stepping stones to the supreme love.

Devotion is likewise incomplete when love exists only for the formless, transcendent God. Love must also rise to embrace all forms—the immanent God. Religionists develop love to its highest level by learning to perceive the Divine in all creation and experiencing all creation as worthy of love. Until then, supreme love has not been attained.

Supreme love is love for everything and everyone at all times. It is a love that gives without limit and receives without limit. One sees God everywhere and loves what he sees, and one feels himself a part of God and accepts the love of the Divine. To seek to always love and be loved—can there be a more worthy and rewarding goal?

अमृतस्वरुपा च ।

amṛtasvarūpā ca

amṛta—*nectar of immortality*
svarūpā—*essence*
ca—*and*

Verse 3:
And its essence is the nectar of immortality.

This verse, a continuation of the previous one, describes the essence, or natural state, of spiritual devotion. Here Narada uses the term *amṛta [amrita]*, literally "nectar," to describe divine love. This nectar is described in the yogic tradition as being a subtle energy that the yogi imbibes in a state of

God-communion. The Tibetans refer to amrita as "the supreme medicine" that heals the illness of separative existence.

The use of this term is notable in relation to the aims of other yogic paths. The goal of both jnana yoga and raja yoga is generally stated as *mukti,* "liberation," or *kaivalya,* "isolation." These terms imply freedom or liberation from the worldly existences that cause suffering. An emphasis is placed on allowing one to reside in one's true spiritual Self, transcendent to and isolated from transitory forms. Nature, even all manifestation, is seen as an external bondage from which the yogi seeks to escape.

Amrita, on the other hand, conveys a mood of more positive affirmation. There is no reference to transcendence or isolation, to stony asceticism or dry detachment. Rather, *amrita* communicates a sense of enrichment, nourishment, and delight.

Those familiar with mythology will recognize in this verse an allusion to the quaffing of the alchemical nectar that provides immortality. Drinking the nectar transforms the human being into a divine being. The son of man becomes a son of God. The world is also transformed in the perception of the yogi: the vision of the kingdom of God becomes a reality. All that is finite is seen in the light of the infinite, and thereby its significance is known.

This enlightenment carries with it a continual yearning for more and more devotion, as well as a delight in sharing joy and love with others. As the nature of a tall tree is to generate seeds that may produce other trees, a *bhakta* enjoys sharing devotional practices with other divine lovers, invoking the energy of God-consciousness in increasingly powerful waves.

यल्लब्ध्वा पुमान् सिद्धो भवति अमृतो
भवति तृप्तो भवति ।

yallabdhvā pumān siddho bhavati amṛto bhavati tṛpto bhavati

yat—*that [spiritual devotion]*
labdhvā—*obtaining*
pumān—*man (here, "a person")*
siddhaḥ—*perfect (here, "perfected one")*
bhavati—*becomes*
amṛtaḥ—*nectar of immortality (here, "beyond death")*
bhavati—*becomes*
tṛptaḥ—*fully satisfied*
bhavati—*becomes*

Verse 4:
Obtaining spiritual devotion, a person becomes a siddha, a perfected one, beyond death and fully satisfied.

This verse begins with the remarkable statement that spiritual devotion is sufficient to produce a *siddha,* a "perfected one." In a document such as these bhakti sutras, terms are used with great precision. Narada uses *siddha* with the deliberate intention of highlighting the potency of spiritual devotion and what might well be gained by the earnest aspirant.

The perfection of a siddha refers to the summation of the evolutionary path of a soul. The indicator of a siddha is an elimination of the root *klesha,* or "bondage," that Sage Patanjali refers to in his yoga sutras as *avidya,* "primal ignorance." This primal ignorance is the false notion that the soul has actually separated herself from God. It is the illusory perception of the wave existing independent of the ocean.

Through an agelong process, the pure consciousness of the soul has identified itself with the myriad forms with which she has been associated. This identification with form results in the soul believing herself to be a limited ego, existing in bondage and suffering. As the ego progresses on the spiritual path it begins to awaken to the recognition that it is not in bondage at all, that it is none other than a soul whose nature is sat-chit-ananda, ever-existing consciousness and joy. The full awakening and stabilization in this consciousness is indicated by the term *siddha.*

In addition, a siddha is one who has obtained *siddhis,* or "yogic powers," powers that provide mastery over the energies of the manifest world in a manner seemingly miraculous to lesser evolved beings. The eight siddhis traditionally cited are referred to in the Yoga-Bhashya (III.45) as:

1. *animan,* "atomization"—the ability to become infinitely small;
2. *mahiman,* "magnification"—the ability to become infinitely large;
3. *laghiman,* "levitation"—the ability to overcome gravity;
4. *prapti,* "extension"—the ability to reach anywhere;
5. *prakamya,* "irresistible will"—the ability to overcome the properties of material elements;
6. *vashitva,* "mastery"—dominion over any aspect of creation;
7. *ishitritva,* "lordship"—mastery over nature;
8. *kama-avasayitva,* "fulfillment of desires"—the ability to manifest all desires.

It should be noted that siddhis are never sought by the true yogi; they simply appear as the result of advanced spiritual practice. Some schools state that siddhis are actually great impediments to final accomplishment. Others hold that siddhis are naturally obtained as a result of great *sadhanas* (spiritual practices), usually involving extreme and dangerous *tapas* (austerities) over the course of one or more lives. In the hatha yoga tradition, for example, detailed accounts of practices that result in specific siddhis are described in both the Hatha Yoga Pradipika and the Gerhanda Samhita.

Other notable indicators of the state of a siddha as indicated by Narada are immortality and full satisfaction. Immortality is the recognition by the soul of her sat-chit-ananda nature. When the soul abides in herself, she overcomes the limitations and suffering inherent in attachment to a body/mind complex. The cosmic drama of apparent separation and reunion with God is perceived in a light of gentle humor, compassion, and playfulness.

Tṛptaḥ [triptaha], "fully satisfied," refers to a state of fulfillment and completion. All karmas have been resolved, and there are no longer harvests to be reaped. All that was once potential has become accomplished. All of the lessons to be learned from the cycle of births and deaths have been finished, and the resulting wisdom and compassion are carried forward by the liberated soul. The purpose of the spiritual path has been fulfilled: God's love has blossomed fully into the love of God.

यत् प्राप्य न किञ्चिद् वाञ्छति न शोचति
न द्वेष्टि न रमते नोत्साही भवति ।

yat prāpya na kiñcid vāñchati na śocati na dveṣṭi na ramate notsāhī bhavati

yat—*that [spiritual devotion]*
prāpya—*achieving*
na—*not*
kiñcid—*anything*
vāñchati—*desires*
na—*not*
śocati—*grieves*
na—*not*
dveṣṭi—*hates*
na—*not*
ramate—*rejoice in fleeting happiness*
notsāhī—*without passion for personal concerns*
bhavati—*becomes*

Verse 5:
Achieving spiritual devotion, one becomes completely desireless—grieving not, hating not, not rejoicing in fleeting happiness, without passion for personal concerns.

Complete desirelessness is not a stoic lack of appreciation for or removal from the world. It is the partner of the full satisfaction referred to in the previous verse. No selfish needs or wants exist in the consciousness of the one who has achieved devotion, so there is no longer feverish yearning. Instead, there exists quiet and peace.

The only desire that remains is to become more fully devoted to God, a desire deemed transcendental by some schools of bhakti yoga. The one who has gained this state and lives without grief, hate, or relative happiness resides in the world while in communion with God. He no longer projects his egoistic desires onto others, viewing them in light of the pairs of opposites (attraction and repulsion), so he can see others as they truly are—pilgrims like himself. This communion breeds in one a sense of community where all are seen as brothers and sisters of the one Father/Mother God.

Accepting the transitive nature of all forms, one lives with the wisdom that everything is impermanent, so there is no disappointment when the natural and inevitable destruction of form occurs. If one lives with the understanding that all that is made of earth will one day return to earth, there is no reason for grief. Seeing a cup as a temporary transformation of clay, one can fully appreciate and utilize the cup, but one is not dismayed when it falls on the floor and breaks.

All hate, enmity, or distaste arise because of selfish desires. Someone or something does not fulfill its role in one's egoistic plans, so it is condemned. The reasons for hate appear to be many, often posing as right and reasonable, but their roots all lead back to the seed of egoistic desire: "I want."

Relinquishing selfish wants, one is free to allow others to travel their own paths under the will of God. One may not like the will of God as it is, but, similar to the useless habit of complaining about the weather, complaining about the will of God is a waste of energy and only reveals our own arrogance. After all, perhaps God's wisdom as to what is best for his creations is more correct than our opinions.

We may consider what Baba Hari Dass has said: "The will of God is not for weak people."*

To be free of fleeting happiness does not mean there exists no happiness; rather, happiness is present at all times as an undercurrent. It is not relative to circumstances. It is the steady rhythm around which plays the melody of life. For the gambler, a sporting event is enjoyable only if his team is winning. For one who has no personal investment, the same game is an interesting drama of skill, energy, and endurance.

Notsāhī bhavati, "without passion for personal concerns," is an interesting phrase. *Notsāhī [notsahi]* means "zealous, overeager, fanatical"—in modern parlance, "uptight." One who is uptight cannot relax and feel his own steps in the cosmic dance. He is always worried about what is right and wrong, good and bad, and whether or not his desires are being met.

One who has personal concerns does so because he imagines himself separate from God, believing he must arrange for his own needs. Actions performed for selfish purposes reflect a mind worried about satisfying personal concerns. Even when these needs are obtained, the self-centered person still worries about protecting his acquisition from loss. The yogi knows that it is not only exhausting to try and provide for himself but it is also a labor based on the false premise of separation.

Worry and despondency are states of mind that arise from anxiety over personal needs. By dedicating one's activities to service of God and the divine plan based on the best of one's understanding, one comes to experience a sense of deep spiritual security. Through spiritual devotion one exchanges the miniscule potency of the limited ego, the personal self, for the almighty power of the One all-pervading Spirit, the spiritual Self.

---

*From a group conversation with Baba Hari Dass at a retreat in Ontario, Canada, sponsored by the Ashtanga Yoga Fellowship in 1994.

यत ज्ञात्वा मत्तो भवति स्तब्धो भवति
आत्मारामो भवति ।

yat jñātvā matto bhavati stabdho bhavati
ātmārāmo bhavati

yat—*with that [spiritual devotion]*
jñātvā—*knowing (here, "realizing")*
mattaḥ—*intoxicated (here, "spiritually intoxicated")*
bhavati—*becomes*
stabdhaḥ—*stunned (here, "overwhelmed")*
bhavati—*becomes*
ātmārāmaḥ—*rejoice in the Self*
bhavati—*comes to*

Verse 6:
With a realization of spiritual devotion one becomes spiritually intoxicated; one becomes overwhelmed; one comes to rejoice in the Self.

The realization *(jnatva)* that turns one from a person of worldly knowledge into a man or woman of spiritual wisdom carries in its wake a natural sense of joy and well-being. One can see that life has a purpose and one gains a polestar by which to travel in the earthly procession. The meaningless twists and turns of a superficial life are now seen through intuitive vision and can be known in their true light, in relation to the cosmic process. No longer does one tread wearily on lanes of tears and despair; one is a pilgrim with a holy destination.

This transformation can at times be overwhelming. The sweetness of devotion fills one's body and spills over in the form of happiness, tears, song, and dance. One feels intoxicated by an unconditional love blossoming in the heart. One's cup runneth over; the quiet presence of God, the Beloved, takes control of the flow of one's earthly life. A feeling of overpowering divine energy sweeps away one's cares, leaving behind an indescribable tenderness toward all living things.

This Beloved, God, the cause of all of this joy, is discovered to be none other than one's own Self. The notions of separation based on false bodily and social identities is seen to be the result of spiritual forgetfulness. The all-pervading unity is seen to be real; all else is created by the function of mind. Like an actor removing the masks of his stage identities, the Self awakens to its own nature independent of the roles it may play in the worldly drama.

It should be noted that firm establishment in the Self is the final step in the development of spiritual wisdom, whereupon one no longer slips into conditioned patterns of identification with egoic existence. Though this stage may seem far away for many of us, even the relative beginner in yoga practice will quickly reap some benefits of regular sadhana: radiant good health, a quieter mind, and a more peaceful heart. As one progresses, the light of the spiritual sun peeks through the clouds of delusion and one enjoys brief glimpses of the peace and joy that are one's birthright. These glimpses inspire confidence in yogic teachings and determination to achieve the goal of Self-realization.

सा न कामयमाना निरोधरूपत्वात् ।

sā na kāmayamānā nirodharūpatvāt

sā—*that [spiritual devotion]*
na—*not*
kāmayamānā—*arising from desire*
nirodharūpatvāt—*the nature of inner stillness*

Verse 7:
Spiritual devotion does not arise from desire. Its nature is a state of inner stillness.

The great yogini Ananda Mayi Ma asked, "Who can be said to be normal in this world? Everyone appears to be mad after one thing or another: some after money, some after beauty, some after music, others after their children, and so forth—no one is really quite balanced."*

It is really very simple. Selfish desire causes one to lose inner peace: the more desire, the less peace. Selfishness causes a fever in the mind, a burning that only becomes stronger when the desires are fulfilled. The fire of selfishness burns all the stronger when the gasoline of fulfillment is poured upon it.

One is often taught in devotional traditions to cultivate one desire alone, the desire to know God. This desire is considered that which negates the pain caused by various other desires. It is likened to a thorn that is used to remove other thorns from the foot and then, itself, is also tossed away. Nowhere in these sutras, however, does Narada recommend the use of such a crutch. In this verse he prescribes a selflessness,

**As the Flower Sheds Its Fragrance* (Calcutta: Sree Sree Anandamayee Charitable Society, 1983), 116. This book is a compilation of discussions with Sri Ananda Mayi Ma.

an inner stillness, that precludes the suggestion of any desires at all.

Turning one's desire system toward the development of devotion is likely a step in the right direction, but the desire for personal benefit is nevertheless quicksand, regardless of its being cloaked in religious garb. Spiritual circles are filled with people who put themselves into postures of devotion because they want to personally enjoy the fruits of devotion. But as Narada here points out, devotion arises not from desires, no matter how "holy," because devotion is itself the control of desires: "Not my will but Thine."

Devotion drives to the heart of an individual's consciousness, below the surface of form and into the essence of content. The mind becomes still, unaffected by external circumstances or internal urges. Mature spiritual devotion requires the relinquishment of all desire, even the desire to personally enjoy the fruits of devotion.

A story from the yogic tradition is illuminating in this regard. Lord Shiva and his consort, Goddess Parvati, were high in their home on Mount Kailas. Parvati reminded Shiva that there were many dedicated yogis who wished to attain enlightenment. She suggested they take a little trip down to the earth realm and see if anyone was deserving.

Shiva was spotted by a group of ascetics who approached him and asked about their chances for enlightenment. The leader of the group told Shiva that he practiced meditation for eighteen hours a day, that he had lived for the past twenty years on fruit only, and that he never cast an eye toward women or money. "Very, very good," said Shiva. "You should be able to attain enlightenment in only three or four more births." The ascetic was disappointed to learn that even after all of his efforts he still had so far to go.

Shiva met with the other ascetics and told them how much

longer they each had until enlightenment—ten lives for one, fifteen for another, and so on. Last, he was approached by a gentle old man who served the group of ascetics by washing their meager clothes and gathering wood for their fires.

He said to Shiva, "Lord, I am too weak to practice any yoga but I try to be a good person. I attempt to serve others and never harm anyone." Shiva, estimating that it would take the man one thousand lives if he continued in this way, did not want to hurt his feelings, so he replied, "Oh, someday you will achieve enlightenment." Unexpectedly, the man began to dance and to sing in joy, "I can achieve enlightenment! It is possible! Enlightenment will one day be mine!"

Suddenly the man turned into a whirlwind of fire that became absorbed into the body of Shiva. Parvati was amazed. "What happened my lord? How did that fellow so quickly become enlightened and fully absorbed in you when those other great ascetics must wait? What special grace did you provide for him?"

"I did nothing," said Shiva. "The ascetics were anxious for the benefits of their labors, so even a few lives seemed frustrating to them. The old man, on the other hand, was overjoyed just to know that he was actually progressing on the spiritual path. His faith in my words and his selflessness opened his heart and quickly he became one with me."

निरोधस्तु लोकवेदव्यापारन्यासः ।

nirodhastu lokavedavyāpāranyāsaḥ

nirodhaḥ—*inner stillness*
tu—*but [related to the previous sutra]*
lokavedavyāpārasya—*performance of worldly and traditional social duties*
nyāsaḥ—*consecration*

Verse 8:
This inner stillness consecrates the performance of worldly and traditional social duties.

In a state of inner stillness, activities undertaken in the world lose their selfish dimension and become consecrated; they become means of expressing Spirit. *Loka-veda* should be understood to mean all activities in the realms of the world—business, political, and social—as well as activities in what we may think of as religious spheres—ethical, familial, and philanthropic works. What is significant in devotional service is not the activity itself but the intention behind the act.

In the Bhagavad Gita, Krishna tells Arjuna that God is most pleased with a simple, sincere offering of a leaf or a piece of fruit (IX.26). When originally written, this was a radical departure from the common belief in India in the necessity of various complex rites believed essential for spiritual development. The Bhagavad Gita and Narada refer to the principle that what makes an activity spiritual is not so much the activity itself but the love that it may express. And love can only be expressed when the mind is still. As Baba Hari Dass once told me, "Love is a state of mind that does not change."

This aphorism points to performing the duties that naturally befall one in the course of life while keeping one's vision on the polestar of God. Renunciation of worldly and societal activities is not called for; what is called for is the transformation of these acts from ego-based to God-based activities, from actions that generate karma to those that manifest dharma. This can only occur in a mind free from the push and pull of likes and dislikes.

तस्मिन्ननन्यता तद्विरोधिषूदासीनता च ।

tasminnananyatā tadvirodhiṣūdāsīnatā ca

tasmin—*in that [inner stillness]*
ananyatā—*single-hearted*
tadvirodhiṣu—*antagonistic to that [spiritual devotion]*
udāsīnatā—*disinterest*
ca—*furthermore*

Verse 9:
Inner stillness, furthermore, requires a single-hearted intention, and disinterest in what is antagonistic to spiritual devotion.

For people without a spiritual orientation, life is a bevy of activity that turns hither and yon with no unifying thread. This is true even for one who develops a purpose in life related to family, career, or adventure of some type. Even the most relatively noble or exciting of these temporal activities will prove dissatisfying because their reward is, ultimately, limited. Furthermore, because the goals themselves are finite, likewise will be the enthusiasm and desire. It is a beautiful fact of nature that no one can eternally maintain ambition for that which is not eternal.

The resolution for the frustration of limited drives and rewards is the transformation of all motivation into a single-hearted devotion to God and the evaluation of undertakings in relation to the furtherance or hindrance of this goal. Upon first mention this may sound like a tremendous undertaking to the novice, but the development of devotion is such that the process is generally gradual and natural, like all of nature's processes. The unification of motives occurs as the result of one's continuing enjoyment of the peace and joy arising from devotion. It may seem like a great undertaking to blanket the earth with snow, but each snowflake falls from the sky in a graceful, effortless descent, unconcerned with the result of its tenure once it reaches the ground.

Udāsīnatā [udasinata], "disinterest," is used in contradistinction to a word meaning "renunciation," which one might expect to find. This indicates the natural manner in which those aspects of life that support suffering for oneself and others—selfish, ego-based aspects—lose their flavor once one tastes the sweetness of love of God.

This is no poetic fancy. Many who begin yoga practice with deep-rooted stress, neuroses, and addictions discover themselves letting go of these past burdens because they discover something that they enjoy more—their true Self. Most people are unhappy because they don't like being who they are. At the same time, it is extremely difficult to renounce pleasure without having a substitute. If one's life is so unsatisfying that an unhealthy activity brings a shred of happiness, it is nigh impossible to give it up unless something that brings greater happiness can be enjoyed in its stead.

A parable may be illuminating. A lion cub was left on its own when its parents were killed. The cub got caught up with a flock of sheep and lived with them, developing all of their habits. One day while hunting, a great lion saw the cub with the sheep and asked why he was living with them. Why was he leading such a limited life when, after all, he was the king of the jungle?

The cub didn't understand what the lion was saying, so the lion took him to a water hole and had him look at his reflection. The cub was astonished to find how strong and beautiful he was. Then the lion demonstrated to the cub how to roar. At first the cub could only emit squeaky growls, but before long he was roaring away. He then happily left the sheep and went to live the full life that was his birthright.

अन्याश्रयाणां त्यागोऽनन्यता ।

anyāśrayāṇāṃ tyāgo'nanyatā

anyāśrayāṇāṃ—*otherwise seeking security*
tyāgaḥ—*relinquish*
ananyatā—*single-hearted*

Verse 10:
When one is single-hearted, one relinquishes seeking security in anything other than God.

Narada here expounds on the first part of the ninth verse concerning single-hearted devotion. Everyone longs for a feeling of safety and support, a knowledge that there exists a safety net beneath him that will provide the resources and nurturing needed during times of trial. This is the whole idea of saving money "for a rainy day," that times of financial hardship may be met with a well of resources. Likewise, human beings are social animals and instinctively seek community—for birds of a feather flock together—so their values and ideals can be confirmed and reinforced.

Narada recognizes the innate human need for support, yet he suggests that the yogi relinquish his dependency on all forms of support other than God. By basing his security on the foundation of single-hearted devotion, the yogi will no longer need the external resources or circumstances that once provided him with a feeling of security.

Even from a strictly practical point of view this makes perfect sense. Temporal forms of support—money, power, friends and family—all come to an end. And when this end will be is an unknown factor, providing an additional, underlying anxiety. As well, the psychological process of dependency breeding contempt comes into play, and an individual is eventually confronted with the deep-rooted fear and hatred that lies at the core of all dependent relationships.

Narada does not suggest eliminating relationships or duties from our lives; he simply proposes that they not be relied upon to provide satisfaction. A social life can be very important, but it is not a substitute for a spiritual life. By turning within and discovering one's spiritual nature, one is no longer placed in a position of weakness and addiction, dependent upon externals for a sense of safety and security. One knows that within there lies a spring from which his thirst can be quenched.

By losing dependency on externals, one develops real compassion and love. One can allow others to be who they truly are because his self-satisfaction is established regardless of whether his affection is returned or not. Likewise, externals can be enjoyed when they are present and easily relinquished when the time of their possession comes to an end because they have not been given a value that they do not have. In this way the yogi lives in the world but is not of it. He enjoys the opportunity to meet and mingle with others and he appropriately utilizes resources as they naturally come his way for the furtherance of God's evolutionary plan.

लोकवेदेषु तदनुकूलाचरणं
तद्विरोधिषूदासीनता ।

lokavedeṣu tadanukūlācaraṇaṃ
tadvirodhiṣūdāsīnatā

lokavedeṣu—*in worldly and traditional social duties*
tadanukūlācaraṇaṃ—*conduct supportive of that [spiritual devotion]*
tadvirodiṣu—*antagonistic to that [spiritual devotion]*
udāsīnatā—*disinterest*

Verse 11:
Disinterest in what is antagonistic to spiritual devotion means worldly and traditional duties are conducted in a manner supportive of spiritual devotion.

Narada here expounds on the second portion of verse 9 concerning disinterest in what is antagonistic or distracting to devotion. In the eighth verse Narada discussed how worldly and ethical duties become consecrated by the control of selfish desires. Here, on a more positive note, he states that these duties should be performed in a manner that serves to support devotion.

The yogi may find himself at a stage in which all activities not directly related to sadhana are found to be unpleasant or distasteful. Narada here instructs the yogi to continue in the performance of his duties in a manner supportive of devotion. One of the primary reasons for this is so that the yogi may serve as a role model for others who are striving to attain what he has accomplished.

"Whatever great people do, ordinary people will imitate. Thus they set the standards for others to follow. As the unwise are bound by their selfish works, let the wise work unselfishly for the benefit of all the world"* (Bhagavad Gita III.21, 25). The yogi directs his body and mind to participate in worldly and social activities under the direction of God as a loving service for his brothers and sisters. Just as an adult will play a silly game with a small child because it brings the youngster such happiness, likewise will the yogi engage in activities of the world as a means of engaging with others and helping to harmonize their consciousness to spiritual vibrations.

The Mahayana school of Buddhism provides a good model in the *bodhisattva.* The bodhisattva is generally thought of as one who has renounced the fruits of enlightenment in order to remain "behind" and continue to be of service to unenlightened beings. For the bhakta, however, there is no sense of renunciation because his desire is only to be of devoted loving service to his Lord, whom he perceives residing in the hearts of all living beings. As such, his service to others is his joy and delight, carrying no overtones of religious arrogance.

To the bhakta the world is a place of pilgrimage, and all living things are his beloved brothers and sisters who are either celebrating their divine nature or seeking to discover their

---

*My original renderings of Bhagavad Gita verses 21 and 25, chapter 3.

divine nature. Either way, his response toward them is, in essence, the same—loving celebration with those of realization, and loving service for those who are struggling. The devotee sees the world as "a carnival of joy," to borrow a phrase from Ramakrishna Paramahamsa, in which he and his Beloved can engage in loving pastimes.

When the yogi observes that others, due to the pollution of desires and attachments, perceive the world in erroneous, conceptual ways, he then utilizes their worldly settings as classrooms in which he can help them learn the lessons of love. Baba Hari Dass has been a great exponent of the value of play. He often stimulated the undertaking of games, especially volleyball, for many of his sometimes sour disciples. When asked how one should approach a competitive contest (as some of these volleyball games turned out to be) he replied, "Die to win, play for fun"—an apt maxim for the life of a yogi.

भवतु निश्चयदार्ढ्यादूर्ध्वं शास्त्ररक्षणाम् ।

bhavatu niścayadārḍhyādūrdhvaṃ śāstrarakṣaṇam

bhavatu—*let there be*
niścaya—*commitment*
dārḍhyād—*firm*
ūrdhvaṃ—*afterward*
śāstra—*scriptural ordinance (here, "ethical code")*
rakṣaṇam—*maintenance*

Verse 12:
Let there be a firm commitment to maintaining an ethical code, even after the development of spiritual devotion.

In verse 11 Narada enjoins the yogi to use his life for developing devotion in his heart and the hearts of others. Narada now utilizes this aphorism and the next to amplify his point. In this aphorism the author alludes to *ṣāstra [shastra],* traditionally understood as "revealed teachings." In historical practice the shastras of the Indian people were related to establishing standards for proper social conduct.

Narada does not allude to any specific shastra, or particular ethical system, as human ethics in the yogic traditions are always understood to be relative. That is, activities are moral only within the context of place and time. Narada is not supporting any one social code of conduct, but is speaking to the yogi whose character must be noble regardless of time, place, and social mores.

The yogi will generally live his life in harmony with existing social codes. One is reminded of Christ's admonition to render unto Caesar what belongs to Caesar and render unto God what belongs to God. The yogi will not be burdened with tasks related to short-lived social or political gains but will utilize his energies toward the achievement of what neither moth nor rust doth corrupt.

Although the yogi may, in rare circumstances, lead others toward an ethical standard in conflict with existing moral or legal codes, this is most usually the role of the social reformer. The yogi is more concerned with exerting his subtle influence on those persons who are receptive to his vibrations. He assists them in evolving from a life based on imperfect human goodwill to one in which they attune to God's omniscient spiritual will.

In verses 77 and 78 Narada presents the ethical standards a yogi is to follow.

अन्यथा पातित्यशङ्कया ।

anyathā pātityaśaṅkayā

anyathā—*otherwise*
pātitya—*fall*
śaṅkayā—*risk*

Verse 13:
Otherwise, there is the risk of a fall.

Narada follows the previous verse by issuing a warning concerning ethical conduct. Previously he encouraged the yogi to maintain a high moral standard while participating in worldly and social activities for the purpose of setting an example and guiding others. Here he counsels the yogi that ethical conduct is also mandatory for his own well-being.

The term *pātitya [patitya],* "fall," refers to the fact that no individual has progressed so far along the spiritual path that he is entirely free of the danger of reversal. As long as one remains in incarnation, the danger of egoism inherent in embodied existence must be respected. Narada urges the yogi to be on guard against the false assumption of security in his established state.

Egoistic tendencies are so powerful and subtle that many an accomplished yogi has fallen. If a man is climbing a one-hundred-foot rope, he only needs to loosen his grasp for a moment to wind up dashed upon the ground. No matter how high he climbs, he must be wary lest he slacken his attention and allow gravity to overwhelm him. And the higher he climbs the greater his risk becomes.

It may be asked how a yogi who has achieved an exalted rank, perhaps even a siddha, could possibly fall. The elevated yogi, one might think, is unlike the struggling aspirant because he is established in a consciousness beyond temptation of selfish motives. Why, then, would a fall occur?

There are two primary reasons. First, when one achieves an elevated stage, not only does one have access to the joys of the kingdom of God, one also has the keys to the world's pleasure chest. The pleasures to be had by the yogi are extremely heightened by his refined senses, body, and mind. It takes strong will to resist temptations of such a high magnitude. Perhaps those of us who have succumbed to lesser temptations may be able to empathize. Even though the accomplished yogi is beyond benefiting from moral behavior, he is not beyond suffering the consequences of inappropriate behavior. In this way, nature assures that no one progresses far along the spiritual path without high ethics and deep humility.

The second reason a fall may occur is that, when one develops a high degree of devotion, one can cross the line from "childlike" to "childish" if a moral code is not adhered to. A childlike devotee is simple, humble, carefree, and dependent on God. A childish devotee becomes lost in the intoxication of the essence of God behind all forms and loses sight of the fact that, in the world of relativity, good and evil still exist. The devotee may be able to perceive the presence of God in both a glass of juice and a tumbler of poison, but it is the fool who would attempt to quench his thirst with the poison. This verse is a gift from Narada that every serious yogi would do well to hold in mind.

लोकोऽपि तावदेव
भोजनादिव्यापारस्त्वाशरीरधारणावधि ।

loko'pi tāvadeva
bhojanādivyāpārastvāśarīradhāraṇāvadhi

lokaḥ—*worldly (here, "worldly duties")*
api—*in addition*
tāvat—*to that extent*
eva—*only*
bhojanādivyāpāraḥ—*performance of activities essential for supporting life*
tu—*but*
āśarīradhāraṇāvadhi—*sustaining the body from death*

Verse 14:

In addition to worldly duties, one should perform activities essential for supporting life, but only to the extent of sustaining the body from death.

Narada concludes his discussion on worldly activities with this verse, which states that the yogi should view his personal physical existence in the same fashion as the rest of his worldly existence. Activities related to maintenance of his life—eating, sleeping, health care—should be undertaken in the same detached spirit as the social and worldly duties previously mentioned are undertaken.

The egoistic person treats the body as a vehicle for achieving pleasure, fame, and power over others. For such a person, the body is a treacherous and undependable friend because it is never sufficient for the goals to which it has been assigned. Egoistic desires only breed further desires. When one gets what he wants, the result is only that he wants more. As such, the natural tendencies of nature—especially death—are viewed as criminal enemies to be fought against. A futile and demeaning struggle! The body always fails to provide sufficient satisfaction to the ego, causing frustration and anger and resulting in rebirth.

When the body is viewed as a temple of the soul it attains its rightful place in nature's grand design. Because the body is not being used for egoistic purposes, its needs are discovered to be simple and easily met. The body is given the natural food and activity it needs. It becomes healthy and energetic, a capable vehicle for the soul's journey during incarnation.

तल्लक्षणानि वाच्यन्ते नानामतभेदात् ।

tallakṣaṇāni vācyante nānāmatabhedāt

tat—*that [supreme devotion]*
lakṣaṇāni—*characteristics*
vācyante—*described*
nānā—*variously*
mata—*point of view*
bhedāt—*differences*

Verse 15:
There are various descriptions of the characteristics of spiritual devotion due to differences in point of view.

Narada here introduces the next section of four verses, which will describe principal means of expressing devotion. The last of the four will be Narada's own definition of devotion. It may be asked why Narada included the first three verses at all. Why did he not simply and concisely detail his own definition of *bhakti?*

The reason for the inclusion of the next three verses is that they address the various means by which devotees express their devotion. A careful review will reveal that the three verses relate to the three levels of creative activity recognized in yoga: actions (verse 16), words (verse 17), and thoughts (verse 18).

These three levels of creativity represent increasing degrees of subtlety by which all beings express themselves and, here, through which the yogi understands his relationship to God. In the concluding verse of this section Narada offers his own comprehensive description of spiritual devotion that embraces, yet transcends, these levels.

पूजादिष्वनुराग इति पाराशर्यः ।

pūjādiṣvanurāga iti Pārāśaryaḥ

pūjādiṣu—*performance of ritual worship*
anurāgaḥ—*intense longing*
iti—*thus (here, "expressed through")*
Pārāśaryaḥ—*son of Pārāśarya, i.e., Sage Vyāsa*

Verse 16:
According to the son of Pārāśarya, Sage Vyāsa, spiritual devotion is expressed through intense longing to perform ritual worship.

The first of the verses giving various descriptions of spiritual devotion represents the opinion said to be expressed by Sage Vyasa, the son of Parasara, a great sage himself. Vyasa is the name of the author attributed to a vast body of writings in yogic traditions, including the Vedas, the Mahabharata (including the Bhagavad Gita), the vast Puranic literature, the Brahma sutras, and other significant works. The orthodox may believe that one individual, Vyasa, was indeed the author of these works, which span millennia. Others believe that a divine inspiration occasionally possesses an author, who then produces an inspired piece of spiritual work. Such an author may be considered an incarnation of Vyasa.

For our purposes, there is no point in debating beliefs. Narada's intention behind introducing Vyasa is twofold: to generally establish the antiquity of the bhakti path, and to specifically call attention to the manner in which the literature attributed to Vyasa presents spiritual devotion.

That bhakti has a tradition dating back to antiquity is not a matter of debate. Bhakti is mentioned as far back as the Shvetashvatara Upanishad, a composition of the third or fourth century B.C. Calling attention to the establishment of bhakti as an integral element of yogic tradition is a device employed by Narada to remind the reader that he is not stating something new in this work. Further, by writing in the form of a sutra the author remains consistent with the literary style of traditional yogic literature.

It should also be noted that much of the literature attributed to Vyasa presents bhakti in the form of actual activity, hence the term *pūjā [puja]*. The practice of puja consists of formal rites, rituals, and practices undertaken by yogis as means of expressing adoration for God. Narada wishes to begin this section with the presentation of spiritual devotion in its most extroverted form.

कथादिष्विति गर्गः ।

kathādiṣviti Gargaḥ

kathādiṣu—*in discussions [of spirituality]*
iti—*thus (here, "expressed through")*
Gargaḥ—*Sage Garga*

Verse 17:
According to Sage Garga, spiritual devotion is expressed through discussions on spiritual themes.

In this verse the devotional activity of the yogi changes from participation in rites and rituals to engaging in discourses about spiritual subjects. One who has been devoted with his hands now becomes devoted in his mind and intellect: listening, speaking, pondering subtle spiritual topics. Garga is a great sage of the bhakti tradition who, it is believed, travels throughout the cosmos expounding the glories of yoga.

आत्मरत्यविरोधेनेति शाण्डिल्यः ।

ātmaratyavirodheneti Śāṇḍilyaḥ

ātma—*the Self*
rati—*delight*
avirodhena—*perpetual*
iti—*thus (here, "expressed by")*
Śāṇḍilyaḥ—*Sage Śāṇḍilya*

Verse 18:
According to Sage Śāṇḍilya, spiritual devotion is expressed by perpetual delight in the Self.

This verse presents the third position of noted authorities describing the methods of spiritual devotion. In this instance, Sage Shandilya is held out as a proponent of bhakti as an internal phenomenon in which the yogi is immersed in the delights of absorption in his true Self, the *atman*. In the previous two verses the yogi was involved in external activities. Here he finds his satisfaction within himself in a most subtle fashion. The sage here referred to is the author of a noted text on devotion, one more academic and polemic than the present work.

This set of three verses, besides presenting different fashions of bhakti, are presenting other types of yoga. The yogi of verse 16 is involved in external, more pronounced activities and is, hence, a karma yogi. The yogi of verse 17 is involved in intellectual, philosophical activities and is taking up jnana yoga. The yogi of verse 18 is involved in a subtle, internal process of raja yoga.

नारदस्तु तदर्पिताखिलाचारता तद्विस्मरणे परमव्याकुलतेति ।

Nāradastu tadarpitākhilācāratā tadvismaraṇe paramavyākulateti

Nāradaḥ—*Sage Nārada [the author]*
tu—*however*

tadarpitākhilācāratā—*that [spiritual devotion] is sanctifying all activities*
tadvismaraṇe—*forgetting that [the object of devotion, the Beloved]*
paramavyākulatā—*supreme anguish*
iti—*thus (here, "expressed by")*

Verse 19:
According to Sage Nārada [the author], however, spiritual devotion is expressed by sanctifying all activities, and by supreme anguish upon forgetting the Beloved.

The summation of this section dealing with different attitudes toward bhakti is here concluded with the author issuing the final opinion. Narada says that bhakti is the sanctification of all activities, inclusive of those recommended in the previous three verses, and the discomfort that arises when the yogi forgets God. Narada makes a distinction between his view of bhakti and those preceding him, not for the purpose of establishing lines of demarcation, but because he wishes bhakti to be considered fully catholic and integrative, that is, to include karma, jnana, and raja methods.

In traditional Indian schools of bhakti yoga, there are considered to be four levels of worship of God. They are:

1. puja bhava—*worshiping state of mind;*
2. stava bhava—*praying state of mind;*
3. dhyana bhava—*meditative state of mind;*
4. brahma bhava—*mind merged in God.*

The first three bhavas are dualistic, implying a separation between devotee and subject of devotion. Verses 16, 17, and

18 are of this type. In verse 16, puja bhava is inferred, verse 17 refers to stava bhava, and verse 18 presents dhyana bhava. Now, in verse 19, Narada recommends brahma bhava, which includes, yet is greater than, the other three states because it implies oneness with God. This oneness is reflected in, yet not contingent upon, activity.

Spiritual devotion is the magic that sanctifies all activities, not only those considered "religious" but also those that we think of as mundane. Religious rites and rituals only become spiritual when they are magnetized by the energy of love. Otherwise they are simply empty gestures. The degeneration of many religious traditions begins when formal techniques of ceremony take precedence over a deep, personal experience of God. Similarly, the most ordinary activity becomes full of spiritual value and significance if it is used as a vehicle for the development of selflessness and the expression of love.

A story: Two yogis had the unseemly habit of smoking cigarettes during periods of prayer. They decided to write to their guru to ask about how to address their problem. One yogi received his reply and was enthusiastic that the guru had given him permission to smoke. The other was disappointed that the guru had denied him the privilege of smoking.

Confused as to why the guru would give conflicting advice, the yogis compared their letters. They found that they had worded their questions somewhat differently. The first asked if it was permissible to pray while smoking. The guru gave his support to this practice. The other yogi asked if it was proper to smoke while praying. To this the guru responded in the negative.

The latter half of the verse dealing with not forgetting God is not intended as a prescription to memorize a formula of godliness in the same way that one might remember a telephone number or the ingredients in a recipe. It refers to constantly holding a mental and emotional intention to remain attuned to God. The yogi becomes, it is said, as sensitive as an eyeball. In this state he is perceptive of his rapport with God and the pain involved in separation from this harmony. The yogi becomes acutely aware of the disastrous effects on his consciousness when he entertains selfish thoughts or emotions. He recognizes the suffering that incurs when he forgets his purpose in life. He becomes like a tender spring flower, sensitive and exposed.

It is worth mentioning that the pain suffered by the yogi upon losing his harmony with the Divine is not the result of punitive damages inflicted by a vengeful deity. It is, rather, the natural consequence of wrong choice. Small children are often attracted to a flame and may burn themselves before they learn the natural law of fire. Likewise, the evolving ego needs to develop the wisdom that all selfishness results in pain. Any thought, word, or deed that carries the seed of ego will, eventually and without exception, blossom into a pain-bearing plant.

Although this may sound like a harsh rule of nature, as one becomes more attuned to the Divine one becomes aware of how simple it is to avoid suffering. The path of love becomes increasingly broad, safe, and enjoyable. One becomes more confident in his own footing, easily avoiding the dangers off the sides of the path.

अस्त्येवमेवम् ।

astyevamevam

asti—*there exist*
evam—*like this* } *(here, "examples")*
evam—*like this*

Verse 20:
There do exist examples of this spiritual devotion.

This verse serves as an introduction to the following set of verses, which discuss preeminent devotion. It also serves as an assurance and inspiration to the aspirant who wonders if his efforts to cultivate divine love will ever bear fruit. During periods of difficulty or spiritual dryness, called "dark nights of the soul" by St. John of the Cross, it is helpful to call to mind our spiritual ancestors who fought, struggled, cried, and eventually succeeded on the path that we are treading. Like us, they too fought many internal battles, emerging victorious and free from the cocoon of ignorance. Their examples may inspire us when we are distraught over our failures and humble us when we are too haughty about our accomplishments.

It is worth noting, once again, Narada's universal spirit. His use of *evam* in the plural reflects his stance that there are various examples of ideal bhakti, suggesting that there exists no one form of worship that is superior. Each aspirant may utilize whatever form of God is most appealing to him, be it Father, Mother, Friend, Protector, or no form at all. There is no hierarchy of distinction in spiritual devotion. What is important is not the specific manner in which God is worshiped but the degree to which the devotee is filled with love.

यथा व्रजगोपिकानाम् ।

yathā Vrajagopikānām

yathā—*such as*
Vraja—*Vraja, Vrindavan*
gopikānām—*of the gopis*

Verse 21:
Such as the gopis of Vraja.

The *gopis* of Vrindavan were shepherdesses who are portrayed in the Bhagavata-Purana and the Gita-Govinda as being completely filled with love for the God-man, Sri Krishna. Krishna is venerated by Hindus as a full *avatar,* or "incarnation of God." Various stories attest to the mad longing that the gopis had for their beloved Krishna. Taken as factual accounts by the orthodox, these tales may also be understood as parables that relate to the soul's longing for God.

One of the most famous episodes related to this longing revolves around Krishna's playing of his flute on the full moon nights by the river Jamuna. The sound of his flute was so maddening to the gopis, so irresistible, that they would leave hearth and home to dance in complete abandon by the riverside. Further, at the height of bliss each gopi would experience Krishna, the perfect partner in divine ecstasy, dancing with her.

The metaphor here is that once the soul hears the enchanting "music" of God, she will be irresistibly drawn to God from that time forward. The world and society will not be able to hold her back because the intoxication of participating in God's great dance is overwhelming. Once the lion learns to roar he will never again settle for the life of a lamb.

This verse begins with the term *yathā [yatha],* "for

example." It is again important to highlight that Narada does not intend to specify one form of bhakti as superior to another. Rather, he states what is but one example of supreme devotion. There exists a multitude of others in yogic and other spiritual traditions.

In the Indian bhakti yoga traditions there are five attitudes toward God that one may possess. These are considered to be hierarchical by traditionalists, but I believe these bhavas are simply mental attitudes and, therefore, only techniques to cultivate spiritual devotion. What is important is not the technique that is used; the pivotal factor is the love that grows in the individual's heart.

The five bhavas are:

1. dasya bhava—*attitude of a servant;*
2. sakhya bhava—*attitude of a friend;*
3. vatsalya bhava—*attitude of a parent;*
4. shanta bhava—*attitude of a philosopher;*
5. kanta bhava—*attitude of a spouse.*

The devotee assumes one of these attitudes in order to develop a personal relationship with a form of God. What is of the greatest significance is not the particular bhava adopted, which will be specific to the temperament of the individual devotee, but that the devotee begin to harmonize his vibrations to God in whatever form he is best capable of understanding and appreciating. It is actually God who plays the role of both worshiper and worshiped. As Baba Hanuman says in the Ramayana, "From the viewpoint of the body, I am Thy servant; from the viewpoint of the ego, I am a portion of Thee; from the viewpoint of the Self, I am Thyself."*

*From the Ramayana by Tulsi Dass.

The mystery of God's divine play is revealed to one who is prepared to adopt with loving devotion any role he feels called upon to play, while at the same time being capable of transcending all dualistic roles in union with God.

तत्रापि न माहात्म्यज्ञानविस्मृत्यपवादः ।

tatrāpi na māhātmyajñānavismṛtyapavādaḥ

tatra—*there [the highest grade of spiritual devotion, as of the gopis]*
api—*even*
na—*not*
māhātmya—*glory [of the Beloved]*
jñāna—*wisdom (here, "mindfulness")*
vismṛti—*forgetfulness*
apavādaḥ—*reproach (here, "degrading the relationship")*

Verse 22:
Even in the highest level of spiritual devotion, as with the gopis, one should remain mindful and not forget the glory of the Beloved, in order to avoid degrading the relationship.

What is recommended here is that the devotee never take for granted nor become too familiar with his Beloved. In the Bhagavad Gita (XI.41–42) Arjuna apologizes to Sri Krishna for making this mistake; he treated Krishna as a friend, as a charioteer, and failed to recognize and appreciate his divinity. If love is to be true bhakti and not simply mundane infatuation (a difference that will be examined in the next verse), the lover must keep the Beloved at a respectful distance.

The greatness of the Beloved in no way belittles the lover. In fact, it may be said that the lover is actually greater than the Beloved. This translates into saying that the devotee is greater than God. The reason for this is that the pure devotee is so completely unified with his Beloved that there exists no factual difference between the two. One arm may appear to have an existence independent of the other but, of course, both arms are joined through a single consciousness.

The devotee and his Beloved are one and the same. God in the form of the devotee can manifest the reality of union while in the world of apparent separation. The devotee is the culmination, the crown of all life. One may say that the purpose of the universe is to produce great lovers. The universe is a vast field in which great yogis blossom forth as flowers of love.

तद्विहीनं जाराणामिव ।

tadvihīnaṃ jārāṇāmiva

tadvihīnam—*forsaking that [mindfulness]*
jārāṇām—*illicit love (here, "selfish passion")*
iva—*as*

Verse 23:
If that mindfulness is forsaken, what exists is selfish passion.

This verse serves two purposes: as a continuation of the idea begun in the previous verse, and as a transition into a discussion about the difference between selfish passion and true love. Verse 22 says that a failure to keep a worshipful, respectful attitude toward one's *ishtadeva* (form of God) will result in a degeneration of spiritual devotion. This leads to the diluted, selfish relationship with God that is often espoused in self-centered prayer. Supplication to a divine being for the sake of satisfying one's desires is not devotion; it is begging. Performing yoga or other religious activities in order to acquire some boon from God is, similarly, a business transaction—I'll do for you, and you do for me.

Bhakti falls to spiritual materialism when one's relationship with God is for the purpose of personal gain. Even if what is gained is some sort of psychic or spiritual experience, the desire for such is still selfish. The supreme devotion of Narada is for no other purpose than the extending of the love of God into ever greater expanses. This love has absolutely no purpose, and because of this it is called mysterious by theologians. To the devotee, however, love is not a mysterious function. Love is the root of all creation, all being, all phenomena, and that which is beyond creation, being, and phenomena. Love is the very essence of God both within and beyond manifestation.

The second aspect of this verse reflects upon the manner in which one relates to other living beings. Bhakti, or "devotion," is no different from *prema,* or "love." We do not truly love because our minds are twisted by desires and repulsions. If we are honest we will recognize that we do not love anyone unconditionally, without reserve and with full commitment. Honoring this truth is humbling, and is the beginning of the purification of the mind necessary for love—true love—to be experienced.

At the core of all relationships between living beings is love, for all beings share the source of love, or God, as their essence. This supreme love becomes colored by the desires and repulsions in the mind and intellect in the same way that clear water becomes colored when powdered dye is poured in it. If the dye can be filtered out, what remains is again pure water. Our egoistic identities arise as a result of the different combinations of colors that dye the pure water of consciousness in each individual.

नास्त्येव तस्मिन् तत्सुखसुखित्वम् ।

nāstyeva tasmin tatsukhasukhitvam

na—*not*
asti—*there is*
eva—*only*
} *there is not only (here, "independent")*

tasmin—*in that [selfish passion]*
tat—*that [the other, the Beloved]*
sukha—*happiness*
sukhitvam—*personal happiness*

Verse 24:
In selfish passion, one's personal happiness is independent of the happiness of the Beloved.

This verse points out that in selfish passion one's own satisfaction and happiness are considered of paramount importance. Concern for one's Beloved or others is not taken wholly into account. The satisfaction of one's desires is the determining factor of happiness and does not consider the welfare of the greater whole.

This selfishness is a cloud of misery that rains on the selfish one and those to whom he relates. Only by selfishness could one participate in any action that would intentionally bring sadness or pain to another. The more one engages in selfish passion, the more one becomes trapped in a quagmire of negative karmic bonds and *samskaras* (thought patterns). The result, the natural consequence, is that one continues to feel alienated and separate from God, which is the very condition of egohood.

सा तु कर्मज्ञानयोगेभ्योऽप्यधिकतरा ।

sā tu karmajñānayogebhyo'pyadhikatarā

sā—*that [spiritual devotion]*
tu—*however*
karma—*activity (here, "service")*
jñāna—*wisdom*
yogebhyaḥ—*of traditional yoga*
api—*even*
adhikatarā—*superior to*

Verse 25:
Spiritual devotion is superior even to the paths of service, wisdom, and traditional yoga.

Here Narada accentuates his opinion as to the supremacy of bhakti as a spiritual path, greater even than the other major yogic traditions: karma yoga, the yoga of active service; jnana yoga, the yoga of intellectual discrimination; and raja yoga, the yoga of meditation and austerity.

On first reading this verse may appear as a sectarian statement, but it is included for two reasons. The first is that bhakti, from a particular point of view, is, indeed, superior to other paths. The nature of this perspective will be outlined in verses 26–33. The second reason is that a practitioner of any spiritual path must have complete confidence that his adopted path is, for him, superior to all others. He must respect other paths, but he must also be fully faithful and absolutely committed to his chosen path. A man who digs many small wells will waste his time, while the man who digs deeply in one spot will find water. A drowning man will fall under if he is indecisive about which life preserver to grab, or if he is constantly exchanging one for another. He must grab a life preserver, cling to it with all his might, and use its buoyancy to help him swim to his goal of safety.

There is no sense arguing that one spiritual path is higher or better than another. In fact, different paths simply take different orientations for their starting points and will naturally describe the resulting experiences differently. If I climb a mountain from the northern trail and you climb it from the southern, we will have very different experiences but we will certainly meet at the same peak. All yogic paths agree that the goal of yoga is some sort of experience of the Divine, of sat-chit-ananda—eternal being, consciousness, bliss. The different paths of yoga are equally valid, providing various opportunities for yogis of different temperaments.

Simplistically it may be said that one of an intellectual temperament will be attracted to jnana yoga, which orients the yogi toward the experience of sat (eternal being, truth). One who is vigorous and energetic will be attracted to raja yoga, leading to an experience of chit, the one consciousness uniting all beings. One of an emotional temperament will be attracted to bhakti and an experience of ananda (bliss, or divine love). But, as discussed in the first verse, since bhakti is essential for the fulfillment of both jnana yoga and raja yoga, it is essential that all spiritual practitioners keep devotion as an undercurrent on their path.

Since *sat-chit-ananda* is only a means for describing an ineffable, inseparable whole, it is incorrect to isolate these aspects from one another. Similarly one cannot describe the sun's attributes as being of light, heat, and energy; the sun does not exist without these qualities, nor do they exist separate from the sun. In the same way the yogi, no matter what his path, will reach his goal and experience sat-chit-ananda as a complete whole.

फलरुपत्वात् ।

phalarūpatvāt

phala—*fruit*
rūpatvāt—*the nature of*

Verse 26:
The nature of these paths is to produce the fruit of spiritual devotion.

Karma yoga, jnana yoga, and raja yoga all have a goal toward which the aspiring yogi is working. Regardless of specific terminology—be it called enlightenment, liberation, or realization—the principle of seeking a goal is present before the student. No matter that these yogis seek an exalted goal; the dynamic of seek, strive, and achieve produces results.

These schools of yoga state that their goals are transcendental to mundane affairs and that they produce no karma.

The fact remains, however, that the students of these types of yogas are involved in the cultivation of fields of experience. As such, they plant seeds and later harvest the fruits. Narada does not criticize this dynamic; he simply points it out.

Implicit in this verse, when seen in relation to the previous verse, is the notion that bhakti yoga is superior to these other yogas because it does not produce fruit (a point that will be expanded upon in verse 30). But if the path of bhakti does not produce the fruit of spiritual growth, the aspirant may ask, why should the determined yogi be interested in these teachings?

The answer to this question reveals the beauty of spiritual devotion. Other spiritual paths require the aspirant to perform strict and specific practices if he hopes to achieve his goal. Likewise, the aspirants are also generally expected to perform service to God and humanity for the betterment of the world. To undertake any activity for a purpose, however, regardless of how noble or elevated, means that one still has a goal in mind. In each of these instances some snake of desire lies camouflaged under the woodpile of spiritual intention.

The bhakti yogi undertakes his spiritual practices and activities in the world with no motive. He does not wish for material gain, nor does he aspire after the fruit of siddhis, or even enlightenment. Love has no reason! Like a spring that bubbles up from the ground, the bhakti yogi finds devotion bubbling from his overfilled heart. He is the most simple of men, finding his natural place in the rhythm of life and gaily dancing. As in dance, no purpose exists; there is no grand meaning, simply the offering of joyful steps and song from a heart that knows of love.

ईश्वरस्याप्यभिमानिद्वेषित्वात्
दैन्यप्रियत्वात् च ।

Īśvarasyāpyabhimānidveṣitvāt dainyapriyatvāt ca

Īśvarasya—*of the Lord*
api—*also*
abhimānidveṣitvāt—*repulsed by egoism*
dainyapriyatvāt—*drawn by love to humility*
ca—*and*

Verse 27:
Spiritual devotion is also superior because the Lord is drawn by love to humility and is repulsed by egoism.

Here Narada introduces the concept of Ishvara, the Lord, and his relationship to the bhakti yogi. Reference to Ishvara is found in yogic writings as early as the Brihad-Aranyaka Upanishad, portions of which may date back to 1500 B.C., as well as in many of the Vedanta-influenced schools. In these contexts Ishvara is generally used in an impersonal sense, referring to a transcendental Self that governs the cosmos and individuated beings.

It is Patanjali who first makes reference to Ishvara in a manner relevant to these bhakti sutras. Patanjali refers to Ishvara as the first guru, the first teacher of spiritual philosophy. Ishvara is considered to be the root guru of all yogic teachings.

Theological exegeses have tried to define and specify Ishvara's status in this regard but, because they were written under the influence of intellectual conjecture, they are not reliable.

Ishvara is an impersonal spiritual energy as well, and a personal presence who can be realized by the yogi. When the universe of illusion first became manifest, sat-chit-ananda assumed a role as, so the Sufis say, "the Spirit of guidance." Similar to the Christian teaching of the Holy Spirit, this function of God is as the divine teacher, the savior, the Christ, of those who are in the bondage of illusion.

Ishvara is often experienced and referred to in a personal sense for two reasons. First, as the ego experiences himself in a personal context, so too will be his initial experiences of God. Later, when the soul transcends egoic identity, likewise will the transcendental nature of Ishvara be realized. The second reason that Ishvara is generally referred to in a personal sense is that this Spirit of guidance becomes manifest through enlightened human beings. As Jesus is considered by Christians to be a manifestation of the Holy Spirit, it can be said that enlightened men and women are manifestations of Ishvara.

Ishvara is drawn to the aspiring bhakti yogi because the bhakta creates a dynamic spiritual magnet by the love in his heart. Grace may appear to be unreliable, but Ishvara does not play favorites. It is a simple law of nature that God is drawn to the devotee by his selflessness and humility. When the yogi creates a vacuum of egolessness, Ishvara fills the empty space with the energy of spiritual guidance. Ramakrishna was fond of saying that the winds of grace are always blowing; one must raise his sail in order to feel their effects.

तस्याः ज्ञानमेव साधनमित्येके ।

tasyā jñānameva sādhanamityeke

tasyāḥ—*its [spiritual devotion]*
jñānam—*wisdom*
eva—*solely*
sādhanam—*means of development*
iti—*thus (here, "assert")*
eke—*some*

Verse 28:
Some assert that spiritual devotion can be developed solely by wisdom.

One of the most influential schools in Indian philosophy at the time these bhakti sutras were written, as well as today, belongs to the Shankara-influenced schools of Advaita Vedanta, absolute nondualism. Shankara is one of the seminal figures in Indian spirituality, living sometime in the seventh or eighth century A.D. He was a brilliant logician and prolific writer who authored commentaries on the principal works of the Vedanta schools during his brief life span of supposedly thirty-three years. In addition he traveled throughout all of India, establishing four principal centers for the dissemination of his teachings, centers that continue to thrive to this day.

Shankara is known as a strict jnana yogi and, although some of his poetry can be seen to reflect inclinations toward bhakti, his writings represent a strict orientation toward jnana. Shankara said that Brahman, an impersonal Absolute, was the only reality. The world and all phenomena, even a personal God, were all illusory.

Many schools that follow Shankara believe that wisdom, and only wisdom, is of any value for the aspirant. These philosophies hold that practices that are oriented toward any function other than Neti, neti ("not this, not this") are, at best, terribly inferior. They hold that bhakti, then, is an optional by-product of jnana.

Narada mentions this belief because he wishes to present a comprehensive portrait of the nature of bhakti, so he must indicate influential contrary opinions and issue a response.

अन्योन्याश्रयत्वमित्येके ।

anyonyāśrayatvamityeke

anyonyāśrayatvam—*mutual dependence (here, "both necessary")*
iti—*thus (here, "assert")*
eke—*some*

Verse 29:
Some assert that wisdom and devotion are both necessary.

Continuing the exploration of opinions that question the power or relevance of bhakti, Narada here makes reference to Vishishta Advaita, qualified nondualism. The founder of this school of thought, Ramanuja, is said to have lived between A.D. 1017 and A.D. 1137. He is best known for his sharp intellect and his criticism of Shankara's absolute nondualism. Ramanuja's principal teaching is that the Absolute is not merely impersonal, but includes itself in the world. Ramanuja rejected Shankara's assertion that the world is illusory; rather, he taught that the world is the body of the Divine.

Ramanuja taught that Ishvara is a personal God who is the basis of the universe. Everything is dependent on God, but free will also exists for individual souls. A soul can turn toward or away from God depending on how she uses her free will. For Ramanuja, bhakti arises from jnana, being the proper use of free will.

This orientation is closer to the pure feeling of devotion that Narada details in the following verses.

स्वयं फलरुपतेति ब्रह्मकुमारः ।

svayaṃ phalarūpateti Brahmakumāraḥ

svayaṃ—*of itself*
phalarūpatā—*reappearance as fruit*
iti—*thus*
Brahmakumāraḥ—*son of Brahmā [Nārada]*

Verse 30:
According to the son of Brahmā, Nārada, spiritual devotion is its own fruit.

Narada here introduces himself and his conclusion as to the relationship of bhakti to jnana. Narada identifies himself as the son of Brahma, God the Creator. It is held in yogic cosmology that when Brahma created the universe he created a few souls directly from his own consciousness, a sort of cosmic immaculate conception. These "children" of Brahma were created as liberated souls and have never participated in any evolutionary sojourn. Their role is to serve as representatives of Ishvara, the Spirit of guidance, in directing and assisting bound egos. The author describes himself as such in order to amplify the significance of these teachings for bhakti.

Narada alludes to verse 26, in which he refers to other yogic paths as being fruit-bearing. Here he explicitly states that bhakti is its own fruit; it serves no secondary purpose, being complete and full in itself. Such is the grandeur of love that it seeks no purpose other than the continued expansion of itself. Pure devotion contains no subtle longing for personal acquisition.

A yogi who is seeking or striving must do so because he feels within himself some sort of lack. Psychologically, the individual feels himself to be less than whole and therefore seeks something or someone to fill his emotional emptiness. Spiritually he is still under the illusion that he exists as an entity separate from God, a wave separate from the ocean.

Narada simply points out the selfless nature of the bhakti yogi. He is not involved in endeavors or pursuits because all that he does is the result of love. He acts not from illusion nor from duty. From the joy and gratitude that he feels as love from God within, his actions spontaneously arise as compassionate service toward the universe and all sentient beings.

राजगृहभोजनादिषु तथैव दृष्टत्वात् ।

rājagṛhabhojanādiṣu tathaiva dṛṣṭatvāt

rājan—*king*
gṛhaṃ—*home*
bhojanādiṣu—*food, etcetera*

tathaiva—*the same as (here, "for example")*
dṛṣṭatvāt—*it is seen*

Verse 31:
This is seen in the examples of a king, home, food, and so forth.

This verse serves as an introduction to the following verse, in which the examples given here are cited as metaphors for the lack of completion that knowledge alone provides. The reason that this verse is included separately is that these verses were originally intended to be memorized and, therefore, it was essential that they be kept brief. This is the general nature of all yogic writings presented in the sutra form, although longer verses are occasionally used for significant purposes (as we shall see later in this text).

न तेन राजा परितोषः क्षुच्छान्तिर्वा ।

na tena rājā paritoṣaḥ kṣucchāntirvā

na—*not*
tena—*by that [wisdom]*
rājā—*royalty*
paritoṣaḥ—*satisfaction*
kṣucchāntiḥ—*appeasement of hunger*
vā—*or*

Verse 32:
Not by wisdom is one made royalty, is one satisfied, or is hunger appeased.

A learned man wished to cross the swollen river, so he engaged the services of a humble ferryman. While crossing, the learned man asked his employee if he had any knowledge of economics and investment. The ferryman replied that he was a man of simple means; he did not have the resources to be involved in financial matters.

"Pity," replied the learned man, "for without knowledge of economics a man is less than complete. I'd say you have wasted a quarter of your life."

After a period of quiet, the learned man asked the ferryman if he had much knowledge of politics. The ferryman apologized and explained that he was busy with his own small family and village; he did not have the time to develop educated opinions regarding such worldly matters. "Pity," the learned man again replied, "for without a knowledge of politics a man is less than complete. I'd say you have wasted half of your life."

The ferryman was paddling his craft when the learned man asked about his knowledge of philosophy. The ferryman replied that he was very busy with caring for his boat and other tools; he did not have the leisure to pursue matters sublime to the mind. "Pity," the learned man replied, "for without a knowledge of philosophy a man is less than complete. I'd say you have wasted three-quarters of your life."

Suddenly, a strong wind toppled the boat and both men were thrown into the water. "Swim toward the shore," the ferryman yelled to his passenger. "I never learned to swim," cried the learned man as he was swept under by the current.

"Pity," thought the ferryman. "He wasted his whole life."

No amount of knowledge is sufficient to provide one with an intimate experience of life's realities. A picture of fire cannot heat a home and reading a book about a foreign land is not the same as actually traveling there. Living by the water and never learning to swim leaves one a stranger in one's own land and a puppet before fate. Narada uses the examples of royalty, satisfaction, and hunger to point out that, no matter how extensive one's learning may be on any of these subjects, it does not provide the individual with the experience itself.

तस्मात् सैव ग्राह्या मुमुक्षुभिः ।

tasmāt saiva grāhyā mumukṣubhiḥ

tasmāt—*therefore*
sā—*that [spiritual devotion]*
eva—*only*
grāhyā—*worthy of being attained*
mumukṣubhiḥ—*those who aspire to liberation*

Verse 33:
Therefore, those who aspire to liberation regard spiritual devotion as the only goal worth attaining.

Here Narada concludes the series of verses that compare knowledge and devotion. He issues a decided opinion about the priority that devotion need hold for the sincere spiritual aspirant. As previously discussed, this opinion is not intended as a sectarian judgment; rather, it is offered to encourage the determined yogi and provide guidance for the confused.

When one places devotion as the polestar before one's path, the light from that star makes life's byways clear and understandable. Most people go through life confused and unsure, never really knowing what they want or where their lives are heading. The yogi intent on cultivating devotion is able to unify his aspirations, placing only the spiritual goal before him.

In this way the accomplished yogi benefits on the physical, emotional, and mental planes. Physically, he does not waste his energy on frivolous pursuits that would leave him drained. By avoiding the superficial in life he becomes a person of great vitality and dynamism, able to realize his goals and manifest his visions.

Emotionally, the yogi is not tossed about by moods and uncertainties because the flame in his heart uses only the oil of devotion for fuel. The yogi does not seek the treasures that moth and dust doth corrupt. He is content and happy living his own autonomous life.

Mentally, the yogi is the strongest among thinkers because his mind is not diluted with a multitude of petty thoughtwaves. He is a man of vision who is aware of what he wants and how to proceed to succeed. He follows the guidance of God and is not distracted in his mind. He knows who he is and what purpose he is to fulfill while on this earth.

तस्याः साधनानि गायन्त्याचार्याः ।

tasyāḥ sādhanāni gāyantyācāryāḥ

tasyāḥ—*its [spiritual devotion]*
sādhanāni—*means of developing*
gāyanti—*sing*
ācāryāḥ—*great teachers*

Verse 34:
Great teachers sing of the means of developing spiritual devotion.

This verse introduces the series of the next four verses, which outline the principal methods by which bhakti is developed. Though various approaches may be recommended by different teachers of spiritual devotion, all of these are to be considered *upayas.* This word is traditionally translated as "technique" or "practice" of spiritual discipline. But *upaya* may also be translated as "a trick." That is, the various methods suggested for spiritual development are nothing more than devices for tricking the mind into quieting itself. In this way *maya,* the divine energy of forgetfulness, becomes undone, and the soul remembers herself and her true nature.

Spiritual practices do not provide the yogi with anything he does not already possess; the wave never was or can be separate from the ocean. Upayas are simply means of unraveling the confusion and bondage of egoic existence. They do not *do* anything; they *undo* the damage done by ignorance. A great Zen teacher confessed that all of his teachings were akin to selling water alongside the river.

Of note in this verse is the use of the verb *gāyanti [gayanti],* "to sing." The author intends here to convey the joyous nature of this spiritual path. All too frequently aspirants are under the impression that elevated states of consciousness leave one distant, cold, and somewhat stodgy. Perhaps this is the result of the proliferation of the philosophies spouted by the self-titled "enlightened" gurus who perpetuate dull and frustrating upayas. As God is of the nature of ananda (ever-increasing bliss), how then could coming closer to God result in less than joy? We would do well to consider Swami Sri Yukteswar's words that the death of spiritual ignorance is the death of all sorrows.

It is true that the person of God-realization may not be jolly in the frivolous, superficial manner to which we might be accustomed. Still, he is certain to be among those smiling and laughing. A furrowed brow will not be found on his forehead and his shoulders do not slope under the cares and burdens felt by the unenlightened. Developing spiritual devotion and drawing closer to God leaves one happy-go-lucky and carefree. Baba Hari Dass has written: "The world is not a burden; we make it a burden by our desires. When the desires are removed, the world is as light as a feather on an elephant's back."*

तत् तु विषयत्यागात् सङ्गत्यागात च ।

tat tu viṣayatyāgāt saṅgatyāgāt ca

tat—*that [spiritual devotion]*
tu—*however (here, used as an emphatic article)*
viṣayatyāgāt—*relinquishing objects*
saṅgatyāgāt—*relinquishing attachment*
ca—*and*

Verse 35:
Spiritual devotion is developed by relinquishing objects and relinquishing attachments.

As the yogi progresses on the spiritual path he becomes aware that the world he sees is little more than a projection of his own mind. His own desires and attachments give rise to the forms he believes he perceives out in the world. The abstract

*Baba Hari Dass, *Ashtanga Yoga Primer* (Santa Cruz: Sri Rama Publishing, 1981).

patterns of energy that are the manifest world are given particular concrete shapes when perceived by an individual mind, in the same way that radio waves are transformed into music when tuned in by an appropriate receiver. As different forms of music can be heard based on which radio station is selected, likewise the manner in which the world is perceived is indicative of the level of consciousness of the perceiver.

With this realization, the yogi naturally relinquishes objects and attachments. As he experiences himself as the source of his world, he spontaneously loses the psychological traits of attraction and repulsion. He becomes free of the clinging and fear that we associate with normal human life. He does not seek security in that which will not last because he has passed beyond the desire for pain and suffering that dominates the subconscious of the overwhelming majority of humanity. The yogi does not build his nest on branches that can be known by the senses or the mind; he knows that freedom is found only in the expanse of causeless love.

The relinquishment of the yogi is a consequence of the joy in his life. It is the harvest of his spiritual development. As a fruit falls off the branch in its proper time, likewise do attachments naturally fall from the bhakti yogi. His relinquishment is not a stoic asceticism nor a sacrifice of anything that might bring happiness. Indeed, to the yogi it is the worldly person who performs the most difficult austerity. He keeps himself imprisoned in ignorance and settles for a few shreds of brief happiness when, with sincere desire, the kingdom of God and its riches are here for the asking. People who seek happiness through selfish desires do not ask for too much; they settle for far too little.

अव्यावृत्तभजनात् ।

avyāvṛttabhajanāt

avyāvṛtta—*unceasing*
bhajanāt—*worship*

Verse 36:
By unceasing worship.

Conventional thought would lead one to believe that this verse is recommending a continual process of prayer, ritual, and supplication, believing these to be the ingredients of worship. But let the sensitive aspirant consider, again, that Narada has chosen his terminology carefully. There is a clue in his use of the word *avyāvṛtta [avyavritta]*, "unceasing."

By definition, that which is unceasing is that which never ends, that which is eternal. All processes of religion, no matter how subtle, are activities that have a beginning and an end. This extends from the most primitive ritual to the most subtle mental exercise of the raja yogi. These practices have their roots in time and can never be unceasing. The aspirant must seek that which is eternal if he wishes to experience the consciousness of spiritual devotion on the sublime level to which Narada is guiding.

A further point to consider is that that which is unceasing must also be that which is effortless and tireless. All efforts are performed by an ego and must be done so with a vehicle, a body. And no body is eternal. Likewise, that which is unceasing must be tireless or frictionless because, as the laws of physics tell us, anything that generates friction will eventually cease to produce energy. Narada asks us to find that which is eternal, beyond time, effortless and tireless.

This conclusion should bring relief to the fevered minds

of those who question whether devotion can ever be gained and God actually known. The answer is that experiencing devotion and realizing God is the natural state of the soul. It is only our own investments in that which is not unceasing that prevent us from entering the eternal stream of love. Like a man who complains of a headache but refuses to stop banging his head against the wall, we are our only enemy in the quest for peace.

All of our selfish efforts to find happiness have only resulted in our digging ourselves into a pit of pain. The bad news is that we have created this mess ourselves. The good news is that we have the power to remedy this miserable situation. We need only orient our minds away from selfish preoccupations and toward unselfish, unceasing love. And just as it takes less time to fill in a trench than it took to dig it, it is a beautiful law of spirituality that our efforts at changing our orientation produce joyful results at a rate much faster than the time it took to produce misery.

लोकेऽपि भगवद्गुणश्रवणकीर्तनात् ।

loke'pi Bhagavadguṇaśravaṇakīrtanāt

loke—*in the world*
api—*as well*
Bhagavad—*God*
guṇa—*attribute*
śravaṇa—*listening*
kīrtanāt—*singing*

Verse 37:
While in the world, as well, by singing and listening to the attributes of God.

For love to be unceasing it must be capable of encompassing everything, everywhere. It must be universal across all of time and space, as well as beyond time and space. Here lies the answer to many of the great theological questions. The bhakti yogi experiences everything as being worthy of love, and since his purified mind loves only God, he comes to the realization that God is everything. All debates about the nature of God and the world are resolved in this experience of love as immanent and transcendent, in form as well as formless.

All beings by dictate of creation participate in the manifestation of God's light, which is of the nature of love. Most human beings are like moons at best, reflecting light. The accomplished yogi, however, is like a sun, actively generating light.

The yogi knows that the world is like a shadow of reality; on the external screen of the world are projected the great dramas of mental experiences. The world process is concrete and reflects the egoic drama of birth, death, and rebirth. The spiritual process is purely abstract and expresses the eternal nature of the loving relationship between God and the souls. The yogi is the link, the intermediary, between spiritual reality and the egoic realities of the temporal realms. He is the light that is in the world but not of the world.

Narada instructs the yogi to sing and listen while in the temporal world. *Singing* and *listening* here have esoteric meanings. *To sing* means to participate in, to be engaged with the world process. The yogi is not to sit back like a bump on a log, content with his own enlightenment. He is to joyously participate in the world process and undertake the various dramas that egos undergo in a manner that generates light. The yogi is also to listen, that is, to hear the echoes of God in all phenomena. He is to be aware that the light of love permeates everything, no matter how dense, and that it is his role to acknowledge that light and nourish its presence in the temporal realms.

मुख्यतस्तु महत्कृपयैव भगवद्कृपालेशाद्
वा ।

mukhyatastu mahatkṛpayaiva
bhagavadkṛpāleśād vā

mukhyataḥ—*primarily*
tu—*but*
mahat—*great (here, "great soul")*
kṛpayā—*by grace*
eva—*only (here, "only from, via")*
Bhagavad—*God*
kṛpā—*grace (here, "blessing")*
leśāt—*minute (here, "mere")*
vā—*or*

Verse 38:
But primarily from the mere grace of God via the blessing of a great soul.

Here Narada concludes the series of verses that began with verse 34, in which he described the means of developing spiritual devotion. In this verse he states that the primary means of developing spiritual devotion is through grace. This grace descends from God through the person of a *mahatma,* a great soul. This teaching is consistent with yogic tradition, which states that it is imperative for an aspirant to learn the spiritual sciences from a qualified guru. Narada cites the extraordinary good fortune of one who can attain the blessing of such a great soul.

Narada posits grace as the foremost means of developing spiritual devotion. Even if the aspirant has succeeded in accomplishing the means set out in the previous three verses—relinquishment, worship, and awareness of God in manifestation—his successes remain incomplete in the face of the grandeur that is ultimately to be accomplished. Even the greatest of yogis attains rather little by his own efforts. A common error on the part of novice yogis is to believe that spiritual practices themselves are sufficient for accomplishment.

When I was a young man, I had the privilege of meeting Swami Brahmanada Saraswati (then Dr. Ramamurti Mishra). In front of a group of several dozen people I asked a question that I thought to be earnest, but that the teacher recognized as revealing my arrogance. He called me up to the front of the room and asked me if I could sit in a half-lotus posture. I did so, and he praised me. Then he asked if I could sit in the full lotus. I took this posture, trying to appear humble in front of the group, but actually feeling quite proud of my asana ability. Dr. Mishra then instructed me to grasp my hair, which I did, and to pull myself up off the ground. Obviously I was unable to do so, and he, I, and the audience all had a good laugh. Even though the laugh was at my expense, it was presented in such a kind way that no feelings were hurt. Such is the manner of a great soul.

महत्सङ्गस्तु दुर्लभोऽगम्योऽमोघश्च ।

mahatsaṅgastu durlabho'gamyo'moghaśca

mahat—*great (here, "great soul")*
saṅgaḥ—*companionship*
tu—*but*
durlabhaḥ—*difficult to attain*
agamyaḥ—*unfathomable*
amoghaḥ—*infallible*
ca—*and*

Verse 39:
But the companionship of a great soul is difficult to obtain. It is unfathomable, and it is infallible.

The companionship of a mahatma is, in itself, an expression of grace because it is not a relationship to which one is inherently entitled, nor one that is earned. It is pure, gratuitous kindness on the part of a guru. The guru's energy first attracts the aspirant, then the guru compassionately, but impersonally, pulls him in like a fish hooked on a line. The less the fish struggles the quicker the fisherman can reel him in. Only in this case the fish is not to be mounted as a sportsman's trophy, but released into new, bountiful waters, more wonderful than he could have imagined.

This is not to absolve the disciple of responsibility; rather, it is to clarify exactly what the disciple is responsible for. The ego has created a sense of separation from God. The mind, under the influence of this egoic illusion, operates in a self-contained, cyclic fashion that can only be disrupted by something outside of itself. The highest thought of which the mind is capable is the notion that it is in a prison of its own making and that it needs assistance in order to break free. The responsibility of the disciple is to discipline his own mind so that it is in a state of humility and receptivity to the power of the guru. Anything less means the disciple is not doing his part. Anything more means the disciple is trying to do more than his part. The aspirant must acknowledge his weakness before he can hope to become strong.

Many youthful aspirants are under the illusion that they must seek out their guru. This is a misunderstanding of how a relationship with the great ones is begun. If the aspirant has developed an intense longing for God in his heart, everything he needs for his growth will be provided at the right time. To understand this process, try to imagine the great ones sitting on a mountain top on a pitch black night, looking down into a large valley. Filling the valley are ordinary human beings involved in their superficial and self-centered lives. But here and there lives an individual seeking God. Those beings have a blaze lit in the heart that shines in the darkness of night, serving as an invitation to the ones on the mountain. The task of the aspirant is to prepare himself, and trust that this age-old adage is true and valid: "When the disciple is ready, the guru appears."

When an aspirant wishes to study with a guru, it is his responsibility to respectfully make a request for guidance. This request is spiritually necessary not only because it establishes the proper conditions under which the guru can teach, but more importantly, the guru can now transmit his subtle energy to the student. A chord of love between hearts is created.

Narada reminds his readers that it may be difficult to obtain companionship with a mahatma. There is no way an aspirant can force such a relationship because a true guru is not attached to having disciples. An authentic guru works only to help his students learn that everything they seek is within themselves. He walks a razor's edge between authority and irrelevance. A sincere disciple learns that the outer teacher is but a reflection of his own soul. He walks an edge between personal responsibility and spiritual surrender. A healthy relationship between a competent guru and a mature disciple is a mutually enriching dance of love.

लभ्यतेऽपि तत्कृपयैव ।

labhyate'pi tatkṛpayaiva

labhyate—*is obtained*
api—*even*
tat—*that [companionship]*
kṛpayā—*by grace*
eva—*only*

Verse 40:
Only by God's grace is their companionship even obtained.

When the yogi begins to see his true situation and to realize how insignificant is his personal life, it dawns upon his mind how unnecessary it is that God or the mahatmas take any interest in him. The stars and planets will continue on their course, the earth will continue to spin, and people, plants, and animals will wind on in their lives regardless of the status of the yogi. Although this may seem like a humiliating blow for the ordinary mind, to the yogi it provides a realization of the nature of grace, of love. He sees that it is not his efforts that have attracted a master. It is solely the benevolence of the master who takes upon himself the task of freeing the bound disciple.

The grace of God is expressed in its highest form in the compassionate service that the great souls render unto humanity, and especially to their chosen disciples. As the yogi progresses on the spiritual path and comes to appreciate all that is being done for him by his teachers, he naturally seeks to extend the same loving kindness to others. In this way God's circle of compassion extends into greater and greater expanses, encompassing more and more sentient beings.

तस्मिंस्तज्जने भेदाभावात् ।

tasmiṃstajjane bhedābhāvāt

tasmin—*in that [the grace of God]*
tajjane—*arising from [the great souls]*
bheda—*difference*
abhāvāt—*because of the absence*

Verse 41:
Because there is no difference between the grace of God and those great souls arising from that grace.

As Patanjali points out in his yoga sutras, all embodied souls are under the influence of avidya, a primal ignorance that creates an illusory sense of separative identity. This sense of individuality, which Patanjali calls *asmita,* or "ego," is like a knot around which what we call a human personality forms. It is like a seed, and the body, mind, and likes and dislikes are the trunk, branches, and leaves of the human being.

Ordinary human beings are born under the spell of illusory identity, and the vast majority lead lives of quiet desperation, as said Emerson, ending only in death. The brief flicker of life—with all its disappointments, short-lived happiness, confusion, unanswered questions, and unmet goals—is the lot of all whose foundation is avidya.

Into this mess God sends his thought of union, of freedom. This thought also takes form, and the form it takes are those great teachers who espouse the spiritual sciences. Although the bodies of the great ones are, of course, comprised of the same elements of nature as the rest of humanity, their bodies subside on a vibrational level much higher than the level of ordinary people. This is because the purpose for which they use their bodies and minds are so different, like a knife taken from a killer and used by a surgeon, that their entire being becomes transformed. By the purity of motivation, the body of a great soul radiates a beautiful inner illumination.

तदेव साध्यतां तदेव साध्यताम् ।

tadeva sādhyatāṃ tadeva sādhyatām

tat—*that [grace]*
eva—*alone*
sādhyatām—*cultivate*

Verse 42:
Cultivate grace alone; cultivate grace alone.

Here Narada culminates his presentation of the necessity of grace by providing the aspiring bhakti yogi with direction on how to proceed with his sadhana. He does not advocate strenuous practices, fierce austerities, or long and detailed examinations of metaphysical principles. He simply tells the aspirant to cultivate grace.

Grace is the foundation upon which all true spiritual progress rests. Grace alone is sufficient to untangle the knot of ego. Grace alone is the breeze that cools the fever of separative fear, guilt, and sin. Cultivating grace is the answer to all problems of spiritual and worldly life.

Grace is to be cultivated in the same manner that one prepares a garden. The soil of devotion must be tilled, the weeds of selfishness must be pulled, and the seeds of right intention and prayer must be planted. Beyond that, however, the spiritual gardener must recognize that the harvest remains in the hands of the ones who command the sun of wisdom and the rain of compassion. The gardener must have confidence that these great ones are more eager than he to see the harvest arise, yet that in their vision they understand the flow of the seasons of the mind. As such they are patient and can wait until the time is ripe for the aspirant to receive the fruit of his labors.

In the Indian Puranic literature there are numerous examples of beings who have developed immense powers as a result of yogic prowess, yet remain untouched by grace and, hence, unenlightened. In the Ramayana, the demon king, Ravana, is portrayed as being a highly accomplished yogi whose austerities resulted in his lordship over much of the universe and a boon from Brahma that made him almost indestructible and immortal. Because Ravana felt that his status was the result of his own efforts, because he felt himself independent of grace, he ultimately brought about his own downfall in a foolish and tragic fashion.

Let us be wise enough to recognize that a sense of accomplishment on the yogic path is an egoic state of mind. True spirituality, and its companions peace and joy, are found when the spiritual aspirant recognizes his progress as only a benefit of grace.

दुःसङ्गः सर्वथैव त्याज्यः ।

duḥsaṅgaḥ sarvathaiva tyājyaḥ

duḥsaṅgaḥ—*negative companionship*
sarvathā—*in all ways (here, "fully")*
eva—*only [for emphasis]*
tyājyaḥ—*to be relinquished*

Verse 43:
Negative companionship should be fully relinquished.

These next three verses deal with the issue of negative companionship. Though these verses are frequently interpreted in an exoteric sense as an admonition to remove oneself from society, the more mature student can come to appreciate that Narada actually refers to an inner process of detachment from negative personality traits. Especially as we refer back to verses 8 through 15, we can see that the author does not recommend seclusion. This is because hiding from the external world does not free one from inner negative companions. This is made evident by many who have attempted to isolate themselves in ashrams or monasteries, only to find out that these milieus are often the breeding grounds for ego games and personality conflicts that make the general society seem tame!

The true yogi is a *viraha,* a spiritual hero. He goes forth into the world without fear, looking at the flaws of the world directly and without flinching. He is not afraid of being contaminated by the world and he does not project his inner negativities onto the outer world. He knows the yogic battle is on the inside, and as he becomes victorious he moves through the world in harmony with his circumstances.

The aspirant would do well to avoid those "spiritual teachers" who delight in pointing out the evils of the world. These are immature egos attempting to discard their own negativities by projecting them onto others. The true yogi is one who is like a lion with himself, always striving to eradicate that which shadows his inner light, and like a lamb with others, always striving to see their inner light, no matter how dense may be the clouds that hide it. He is the king of the jungle of his world. He hides from no one and seeks escape from nothing.

कामक्रोधमोहस्मृतिभ्रंशबुद्धिनाश
सर्वनाशकारणत्वात् ।

kāmakrodhamohasmṛtibhraṃśa-
buddhināśasarvanāśakāraṇatvāt

kāma—*selfish desire*

krodha—*anger*

moha—*delusion*

smṛtibhraṃśa—*deprivation of memory (here, "forgetting spiritual goal")*

buddhināśa—*loss of buddhi, the faculty of discrimination*

sarvanāśa—*loss of all (here, "loss of everything worthwhile")*
kāraṇatvāt—*being the cause of*

Verse 44:
Negative companionship is the cause of selfish desire, anger, delusion, forgetting one's spiritual goal, loss of discrimination, and the loss of everything worthwhile.

Contrary to popular Western belief, the mind does not produce thoughts. The mind is, rather, a vessel in which thoughts are held. The particular thoughts held in the mind are the result of decisions made by the *buddhi* (the discriminating intellect). (The nature of mental processes is discussed in greater detail in the commentary to verse 48.) As such, we can appreciate that thoughts are the "companions" of the individual. They are the traveling partners he chooses as he makes his way through life. Narada will examine the result of choosing selfish partners and allowing them to make their home in one's mind.

Narada employs a frequently used yogic phrase—"*kama, krodha, moha*" ("desire, anger, delusion")—to alert the aspirant to the commonality of disaster awaiting all those who allow negativities to exist as their companions. Desire, anger, and delusion reinforce each other and send the aspirant into a downward cycle of pain, depression, and despair.

Under the force of avidya (spiritual forgetfulness) the egoic personality develops selfish desires. Because the world often thwarts the acquisition of his desires, the individual then becomes angry at those he perceives as blocking his satisfaction. Experiencing anger and separation from others, he becomes further deluded, falling into a state of spiritual amnesia *(smrtibrahmsa)* such that he completely forgets his spiritual identity and spiritual goals. The result is that he finds himself in conflict within his own heart, and at war with others in the outer world.

As the individual becomes increasingly involved in this cycle of delusion, the ability of the buddhi to make wise decisions regarding which thoughts to accept into the mind becomes weakened. Like a muscle that is not exercised, the intellect grows flaccid and falls prey to conditions of fear, guilt, and ignorance. Selfish, negative forces take dominance and the individual's life becomes filled with frustration, anxiety, and fear. Life loses its luster and one experiences *sarvanasa,* a feeling of losing everything worthwhile.

तरङ्गायिता अपीमे सङ्गात् समुद्रायन्ति ।

taraṅgāyitā apīme saṅgāt samudrāyanti

taraṅgāyitā—*acting as small waves*
api—*even*
ime—*these*
saṅgāt—*by companionship*
samudrāyanti—*become like a swelling ocean*

Verse 45:
A swelling ocean is raised from the small waves of companionship.

Although the dynamics discussed in the previous verse may sound grim upon first reading, it is important that the aspirant recognize how disastrous is the companionship of negative thoughts. It takes but one step off the tightrope for the circus performer to fall to his death. Narada wants the aspiring yogi to be alert and on guard to the problems that will arise from negative thoughts. Better not to plant seeds of selfishness than try to eradicate them once they have grown into giant weeds.

Narada uses the analogy of an ocean to illustrate the result of negative tendencies. Small waves eventually produce great effects. The wise aspirant will take this warning to heart and be extremely vigilant in not allowing thoughts of selfishness, fear, and guilt to become his companions. Do not allow yourself the indulgence of entertaining negative thoughts!

कस्तरति कस्तरति मायाम् ? यः
सङ्गंत्यजति, यो महानुभावं सेवते,
निर्ममो भवति ।

kastarati kastarati māyām? yaḥ saṅgaṃtyajati yo mahānubhāvaṃ sevate nirmamo bhavati

kaḥ—*who?*

tarati—*crosses*

kaḥ—*who?*

tarati—*crosses*

māyām—*the [ocean] of Great Illusion*

yaḥ—*one who*

saṅgaṃ—*companions (here, "attachment to others")*

tyajati—*relinquishes*

yaḥ—*one who*
mahānubhāvaṃ—*great souls*
sevate—*serves*
nirmamaḥ—*without "I" sense (here, "ego free")*
bhavati—*becomes*

Verse 46:
Who crosses, who crosses the ocean of the Great Illusion? One who becomes ego free, who serves the great souls, and who relinquishes attachment to others.

In a poetic metaphor for the spiritual journey, Narada asks the question: Who crosses over the expanse of the great illusion of separation from God? The source of this illusion, maya, is the energy of God that generates his *lila* (play or sport) of separation and reunion. In orthodox Indian literature, maya is frequently feminized and ofttimes referred to as a mistress of illusion, a cosmic temptress, a sort of female Satan. The bhakti yogi, however, sees that Maya is God's beloved consort. She is the perfection of love, harmony, and beauty. It is she who gives birth to the many from the One. The entire universe is her body. The bhakti yogi loves and respects Maya; by being in right relationship with her, he is in right relationship with all creation.

The first characteristic of the one who can cross that ocean is that he becomes ego free. He loses his sense of separate identity. He remembers his pure identity in God, releasing the illusory sense of self-creation based on physical, mental, and social identities. The acorn on the tree recognizes that it was created in the image of its "father," and that it shares the same characteristics as its father. Furthermore, it is the will of its creator that it too one day become a great and powerful tree, itself producing acorns and thus forever expanding the cycle of life.

The second characteristic of the one capable of crossing the ocean of illusion is that he serves the great ones, the mahatmas originally mentioned in verse 38. To serve the great ones means to take one's own part in God's plan. To truly serve the great ones means to find one's place in the grand dance of life and to then follow one's own calling. Each soul has its own note to sing in the divine chorus and no voice is more important than another. As Krishna tells Arjuna in the Bhagavad Gita, "It is better to follow your own calling imperfectly than follow another's perfectly. If death should come while following your own path, this is surely better than living with the fear and anguish of following a false path"* (III.35).

As we saw before, in verse 8, the essential component in spirituality is motivation, not activity. A task becomes spiritualized to the extent that it is used as a vehicle to express love. Mahatma Gandhi once said, "What you do may not seem important, but it is very important that you do it." There is no hierarchy of activity in the vision of love.

There is a beautiful story from the Jewish tradition that highlights this point. One morning one of the students of Rabbi Zusha, a great lover of God, came to the Rabbi's home and found the Rabbi in tears. The student asked the Rabbi why he was crying. The Rabbi responded that the previous night, during his prayers, he had a vision of God.

The student was awestruck that his Rabbi had personally experienced a vision of God. He asked the Rabbi what could have occurred that such a magnanimous event could

---

*My original rendering of Bhagavad Gita verse 35, chapter 3.

possibly bring sadness. The Rabbi answered, "All my life I have tried to be a good Jew. I have striven to be like Abraham, to be like Isaac, to be like Moses. Then last night, when I spoke with God, he asked me why I had wanted to be other than as he created me. He wanted to know why I had not striven to be like Zusha. And as Zusha is someone I had never really loved, I realize that I have been failing in my spiritual life. This is why I cry."

The third characteristic of one who is able to cross the ocean of illusion is that he relinquishes attachments to others. From a psychological standpoint, he becomes free of clinging to those he likes and of separating himself from those he dislikes. From a spiritual perspective, he becomes free of the selfishness that results in clinging and of the fear that results in separation. Without clinging or fear, the yogi becomes free.

When a yogi experiences freedom, he finds contentment and fulfillment within himself. He ceases to become lost in the social and familial dramas that pose as love but that are actually based on insecurity and immaturity. He stops projecting his inner turmoils onto others; he no longer views anyone as an enemy. All beings become equal in his eyes, equally worthy of love.

यो विविक्तस्थानं सेवते, यो
लोकबन्धमुन्मूलयति, निस्त्रैगुण्यो भवति,
योगक्षेमं त्यजति ।

yo viviktasthānaṃ sevate yo
lokabandhamunmūlayati nistraiguṇyo bhavati
yogakṣemaṃ tyajati

yaḥ—*one who*
viviktasthānaṃ—*solitude*
sevate—*resorts to*
yaḥ—*one who*
lokabhandaṃ—*bondage of the world*
unmūlayati—*eradicates*
nistraiguṇyo—*free of the three modes of nature*
bhavati—*becomes*
yogakṣemaṃ—*concern for acquisitions that provide happiness*
tyajati—*relinquishes*

Verse 47:
One who resorts to solitude, who eradicates the bondage of the world, who becomes free of the three modes of nature, and who relinquishes the feeling that happiness is dependent on acquisitions.

Four characteristics of the one who overcomes illusion are here presented. The first is that one must be capable of resorting to solitude. It must again be emphasized that this solitude is of an inner nature; it does not necessarily relate to external conditions. The aspirant must be able to maintain a solid inner consciousness regardless of circumstances, regardless of time and space. He must be able to keep love alive within his heart amidst, as Yogananda has said, the crash and thunder of "dissolving worlds." Too many yogis have spent years in external solitude, only to realize how fragile was their accomplishment as soon as they again entered the marketplace.

A parable may illustrate the nature of one in true solitude. There once was a criminal who was sentenced to death by his king. The king gave the man one chance to save his life: He must carry a chalice filled with water around the entire circumference of the kingdom without spilling a drop. It took the man several days to accomplish this task. He was always alert, not for a moment breaking his concentration. After the successful fulfillment of this requirement, his sentence was commuted. When asked later what he saw during his journey, he replied that he saw only one thing: the chalice of water.

Our consciousness is our pearl of great price. To spill our awareness on objects and activities that soil our beauty does not demonstrate wisdom. We do well to keep our awareness safe in the solitude of our hearts, protecting it from the ravages of egoic thoughts, bringing it into the open only when its luster can be shared with other lovers of God.

The ocean of illusion is crossed by one who has eradicated the bondage of the world. This bondage is the spiritual ignorance (avidya) from whose seed grows the tree of egoic obstructions. In his yoga sutras, Patanjali denotes the nature of the bondage of ignorance thus: "Avidya is the condition of confusing the eternal, innocent, blissful Self with that which is impermanent, impure, pained, and not-Self"* (II.5).

---

*My original rendering of Patanjali's Yoga Sutra verse 5, chapter 2.

There exist two flows of energy in the realms of manifestation. The first flow arises from the energy of avidya; it entangles the soul in conditions of sin, guilt, fear, and doubt about her true nature and identity. The other flow of energy arises from Ishvara, the Lord, whose energy serves as a message to the soul, reminding her of her eternal, innocent, blissful identity in God. The yogi who can cross the ocean of illusion is one who can discern the difference between these two energies in all spheres of life, from the macrocosmic to the microcosmic.

The bonds of the world have three strands, the three *gunas* or "energies of nature." These are *sattva,* the energy of lucidity; *rajas,* the energy of passion; and *tamas,* the energy of inertia. Avidya is the force behind the operation of these three energies. Rajas is the principle behind all of the selfish motivations that inspire a person into egoic activities. Desires for money, social position, and fame are examples of the influence of rajas. Tamas is the principle behind the laziness and sickness that prevent a person from living in harmony within and without. Overeating, poor health, and lack of enthusiasm for life are examples of the influence of tamas.

Sattva is the principle of balance. Sattva predominates when a person is not swayed by rajas or tamas. His mind then comes into balance; it becomes peaceful. Sattva is the principle behind compassion, generosity, and the desire for knowledge. Sattva is still a binding energy, but it is the life raft that enables one to avoid drowning in the waves of rajas and tamas. When one reaches the safe shore of devotion, one may then dispose of the raft of sattva.

To cross the ocean of illusion one must relinquish the feeling that happiness is dependent on acquisitions. Many religious practitioners undergo austerities in an attempt to renounce objects, but there are inherent problems with this strategy. The one who practices austerity fights against the darkness of dependency, but the more he fights the more darkness he finds to fight against. To fight against something requires a feeling of separation, and separation is the very condition of darkness. Austerity is an endless path of tension and struggle.

The bhakti yogi, on the other hand, allows renunciation to occur as a natural process. He does not fight against darkness; he simply lights candles of devotion to his Beloved. Each candle he lights illumines the darkness, until so much light is ablaze that there is no darkness to be found. If he finds that he has trapped himself in some dependency, he simply laughs at his own foolishness and prayerfully offers what he does not want to God, confident that God will help him release it in glad exchange for the peace and joy that he does want. In this way the bhakti yogi enjoys a natural process of continued spiritual happiness that effortlessly includes releasing dependency on objects. Devotion is also an endless path, but it is covered with gentle grasses and lined with beautiful flowers, and it continually reveals new vistas of grandeur and delight.

यः कर्मफलं त्यजति, कर्माणि सन्न्यस्यति,
ततो निर्द्वन्द्वो भवति ।

yaḥ karmaphalaṃ tyajati karmāṇi sannyasyati
tato nirdvandvo bhavati

yaḥ—*one who*
karmaphalaṃ—*fruit of activity*
tyajati—*relinquishes*

karmāṇi—*actions (here, "egoistic actions")*
sannyasyati—*renounces*
tataḥ—*thereby*
nirdvandvaḥ—*free of the pairs of opposites*
bhavati—*becomes*

Verse 48:
One who relinquishes the fruits of activity, who renounces egoistic actions, thereby becomes free of the pairs of opposites.

This verse presents three additional characteristics of the one who crosses the ocean of illusion. Narada states that such a one relinquishes the fruits of activity. This is the philosophy behind karma yoga, the yoga of selfless service. In karma yoga an aspirant attempts to perform all activities as a duty, without thought for reward or recognition. It is a path that is intended to diminish personal motivations for the undertaking of actions. The ideal karma yogi is one who develops a sense that he is simply an instrument of God's will and that all of his acts in this world are reflections of God's will.

The second characteristic discussed in this verse is that one renounces egoistic actions. It may be helpful at this point to discuss the yogic model of consciousness in order to gain a precise sense of what is meant by *egoistic actions*.

According to yogic psychology, the overall mental structure of an individual human being is comprised of four components. They are *manas*, or "mind"; *buddhi*, or "intellect"; *ahamkara*, or "ego"; and *chitta*, or "substructure of consciousness."

Mental processes take place as follows. The sense organs receive impressions from the energy vibrations of the outside world. The manas, or mind, takes these vibrations and generates a form, a picture of what is then identified as the world "outside." The buddhi, or intellect, identifies the objects pictured and designates them as belonging to general and specific classes. Ahamkara, or ego, passes a judgment on the "exterior" scene, using evaluations based on whether or not it believes the object helps it in its objectives. The chitta, or substructure, absorbs the processes of the manas, buddhi, and ahamkara, recording these in subtle forms known as samskaras, or seeds. These seeds then grow in the chitta, creating the inner promptings that in psychology are called *motivations*.

For example, a man receives sensory data from his eyes and nose that the manas compiles and generates as a picture and aroma of an object. The buddhi announces the mental image to be a fragrant pizza. The ahamkara then decides whether or not the pizza is a desirable object based on its considerations of hunger and other variables. The chitta records this process and the next time the man experiences the biological phenomenon known as hunger, chitta will stimulate the other components of the mind to remember the object known as a pizza and then, via the sense organs, direct the mind to procure such an object.

The process seems benign enough when discussing the mechanisms of hunger and pizza acquisition, but there is an inherent problem in the nature of ahamkara. Ego, by its very design, is a process built on principles of self-preservation, self-expansion, and self-expression, regardless of consequences to others. Ego, as a mechanism, is incapable of empathy or compassion. As Sigmund Freud recognized, it has one mission and one mission only: to obtain pleasure and avoid pain. The ego unencumbered by spiritual aspiration is a pure expression of selfishness, greed, and insatiable appetites.

The yogi quells the ravages of the ego by the practice of

yoga—in this context, karma yoga. By following what he understands as the will of God, the yogi performs actions whether they appear pleasant or unpleasant, in a spirit of detached benevolence. As a result of his advancement in karma yoga, the aspirant gradually dissolves the selfish aspects of ego. The result is that the manas operates in a healthy and efficient manner, buddhi becomes strengthened and matures into its highest capability, and the chitta becomes a reservoir of positive thoughts and inclinations.

Through the reduction of the ego, the aspirant becomes free of the concerns of the body and the limited mind. These are frequently designated in yogic literature as "the pairs of opposites." These include pleasure and pain, fame and disrepute, desire and repulsion. The yogi lives life from a balanced space, neither striving nor avoiding, simply doing what needs to be done. He is the master of his life and is not tossed by the waves of external circumstances.

यो वेदानपि सन्न्यस्यति
केवलमविच्छिन्नानुरागम् लभते ।

yo vedānapi sannyasyati
kevalamavicchinnānurāgam labhate

yaḥ—*one who*
vedān—*the Vedas [religious scriptures]*
api—*even*
sannyasyati—*renounces*
kevalam—*complete*
avicchinna—*unceasing*

anurāgam—*intense longing*
labhate—*is obtained*

Verse 49:
Renouncing even the scriptures, a complete, unceasing, intense longing for God is obtained.

This is a beautiful and striking verse in which Narada invites the bhakti yogi to be free of the bondage of orthodox doctrine. Narada encourages the aspirant to strive for a state of intense, unceasing love for God, heedless even of the demands of traditional and social religious teachings.

Every organized religion holds that certain behaviors, rituals, personalities, places, and/or books are sacred. These organized teachings are proper in their own place, but they are mere options for the one infused with devotion. To such a one, God is direct and spontaneous, providing him with an immediate source of guidance and direction. His relationship with God is not mediated through anyone or anything.

We can refer back to verse 21 and to the reference to the gopis of Vraja as being the highest expression of spiritual devotion. Krishna and his beloved consorts were violators of major social taboos. In his early childhood Krishna is depicted as a thief, as a disrupter of religious ceremony, and as being disrespectful to those of authority. As he grows older he becomes a shameless flirt and a romantic heartbreaker. His irresistible attractiveness leads to amorous adventures with the gopis, many of whom are married, resulting in the disruption of family and community life.

Perhaps these tales are metaphoric, but the point is that heightened levels of devotion free the aspirant from an orthodox and preplanned lifestyle. The bhakti yogi relies not on words or prescribed behaviors to realize his Beloved. Instead, he directly senses the presence of his Beloved within and without, and it is this presence, and only this presence, to which he is obliged.

As the gopis appeared mad before their families and as Christ appeared blasphemous before the Pharisees, the deep lover of God is likely to be misunderstood by his contemporaries. His actions stem from a state of consciousness that cannot be evaluated by the socially based relativities of "right" and "wrong." The devotee does not intentionally violate community standards, but his encompassing devotion sometimes forces him beyond externally imposed rules and regulations. His morality arises from a spiritual vision of the equality of all souls and a deep, all-consuming love for God.

The devotee understands the relative nature of ethics and social codes. Though he does his best to honor them with his behavior, he will not permit the bird of his love to be caged by mere convention.

स तरति स तरति, स लोकांस्तारयति ।

sa tarati sa tarati sa lokāṃstārayati

saḥ—*he*
tarati—*crosses*
saḥ—*he*
tarati—*crosses*
saḥ—*he*
lokān—*all the world*
tārayati—*helps to cross*

Verse 50:
He crosses, he crosses, and he helps all the world to cross.

Here we have the culmination of the preceding set of four verses. The one who fulfills the characteristics described in those verses is capable of crossing the ocean of separative consciousness, and he helps all the world to cross. How he does this is a great teaching, and one that we would do well to investigate.

To examine the issue of how a great soul helps others we must look at the very nature of soul. Ordinary religious people believe every human body contains a soul within it. From an absolute standpoint, there exists only one soul, one conscious Self—God, or sat-chit-ananda. In the spiritual worlds there exists an infinite number of souls, but their relationship to each other and to God is so unified that it is misleading, to those of us in the human realm, to speak of them as separate. To again use the analogy: God is the ocean of eternal, blissful consciousness, and the individual souls are the waves. The waves do not have an existence separate from the ocean, or from each other.

An individual human consciousness is comprised of five *koshas* (sheaths or bodies). These bodies are sometimes said to encompass a soul, but they actually only reflect various portions of the soul's nature and power. They have no sentient existence of their own. These bodies are:

1. *annamaya kosha,* "physical body"—a gross structure comprised of physical matter, such as carbon, nitrogen, and so forth;
2. *pranamaya kosha,* "energy body"—a subtle structure comprised of primal energies that provide the physical form with life force;

3. *manomaya kosha,* "mental body"—a vibratory structure comprised of thought energy, which is thoughts and emotions generated by experience resulting from contact between the mind and the external world through the senses;
4. *vijnanamaya kosha,* "intuitive body"—a more subtle vibratory structure comprised of intuitive energy that reflects insights about the spiritual nature underpinning all experience;
5. *anandamaya kosha,* "bliss body"—a starlike radiance too subtle to be seen or imagined, comprised solely of a reflection of the soul.

All five of these bodies are temporary vessels. The physical and energy bodies relate to the physical world and exist as long as physical life persists. The mental and intuitive bodies relate to the astral worlds and exist for one reincarnational cycle. The bliss body is the dwelling place of the soul, and exists for the duration of the evolutionary sojourn of the soul. But even this bliss body is temporal and distinguishable from the sat-chit-ananda nature of the soul.

The enlightened sage recognizes the unity underlying all consciousness, and he experiences the unity of the souls and God. He perceives forms as temporal boundaries in which bodies and minds only appear to function as independent entities. Individuality is seen to be an illusion. An analogy that Shankara used is that individual existence is like a sealed jar. Air is both within and without the jar. Likewise, the all-pervading consciousness of sat-chit-ananda permeates all animate and inanimate objects, inside and outside, on every sphere of manifestation.

Because of his identity with sat-chit-ananda, the consciousness of an enlightened sage is not bound by any sheaths, even though he may wear a body. The spiritual work that he does affects all beings under the spell of illusion, because those who are fully enlightened experience all phenomena as existing within their own Self. In the same way that your conscious awareness establishes a direct and immediate relationship between your right and left hands, so does the sage experience such a relationship between all supposedly separate beings. He experiences them as limbs united within his consciousness. As he crosses the ocean of illusion, all aspects of his consciousness—the apparently distinct beings—are assisted in their efforts.

अनिर्वचनीयं प्रेमस्वरुपम् ।

anirvacanīyaṃ premasvarūpam

anirvacanīyaṃ—*inexpressible*
prema—*love*
svarūpam—*essential nature*

Verse 51:
The essential nature of love is inexpressible.

The inability of language to express the true nature of love gives the bhakti yogi additional reason for recognizing the restricted value of scriptures. Language, being itself a formulation of the finite human mind, is only capable of expressing aspects of experience that can be recognized and understood by that same finite mind. The love that is infinite exists in a realm beyond the reach of the mind.

This love is an immediate and direct experience that, when mediated through the mind, can only be indirectly alluded to. Even the great works of art and holy scriptures can, at best, serve as signposts to regions beyond their domain. Therefore it is said that before realization, scriptures will be misunderstood; after realization, scriptures will be unnecessary.

Attempting to contain the infinite within the finite symbolism of language may result in scholarship, but it will not produce devotion. At the same time, the enlightened sage recognizes that if he is to share the riches of God with others, he must communicate to them in forms that their minds will recognize and understand. Many great souls only communicate through telepathy, but most ordinary human beings cannot perceive their subtle vibrations. The spoken and written word, then, become mediums of last resort, adopted by teachers to meet the needs of their students. Using language consciously for teaching and contemplation is one method of karma yoga and is a secondary stage of bhakti yoga (see verse 17).

This verse marks the beginning of a section of verse dealing with the nature of spiritual love that continues to verse 55.

मूकास्वादनवत् ।

mūkāsvādanavat

mūka—*mute*
āsvādana—*taste*
vat—*[connotes "resemblance"] (here, "like")*

Verse 52:
Like taste for one who is mute.

This is a most interesting verse as Narada communicates an essential teaching using somewhat whimsical language. We are told in the previous verse that the essential nature of love is inexpressible. Here the experience of taste for one who is mute is used as an example. The example is apt because a person who is mute has no verbal means of describing his experience. He is face to face with the inescapable limits of language and the inability of a human being to directly verbalize experience.

On a more profound level, Narada alludes to a sense organ that is involved in both receptive and dynamic functions—the tongue. The tongue is the sense organ responsible for communicating the experience of taste to the mind, as well as directing the function of speech. Taste is the most primitive of all sensory experiences, and many yoga teachers instruct their students in the disciplines of taste and diet. Mahatma Gandhi was fond of saying that if the tongue is brought under control, the other sense organs will follow.

The second function of the tongue, speech, is among the most primitive means for communication between the inner personality and the external environment. The tongue is a mediator between the inner and outer worlds. It brings in nourishment from the world, making life possible, and it expresses thoughts and emotions, making communication possible. Through this interaction between the inner and outer, the dynamic of personal life is generated and life as an individual human being is made possible.

Relative to our concerns with developing devotion, we must look at the ways in which the tongue can be transformed from a medium of superficial exchange into a vehicle for profound interchange. The key to this lies, as has been previously discussed, with utilizing the body as a means of expressing devotion as opposed to a means of satisfying selfish ego desires. The yogi does not cut out his tongue for fear it might offend; he transforms its functions into reflections of spirituality.

Eating and speaking are two primary ways in which ego-based personalities satisfy their demands. The inability of many people to control their appetite has led to the significant number of diet-related health problems we see in this society, as well as the vast and varied enterprises promoting weight control. The yogi, on the other hand, does not live to eat—he eats to live. By eating a simple and healthy diet he demonstrates how easily health can be maintained.

At the same time, ordinary speech is generally used as a vehicle for expressing attractions and desires, and for expanding the ego's dominion in the spheres of social and family life. The ordinary person speaks as a means of attaining his desires. He often speaks impulsively, and he feels it his right to express angry words when he deems himself justified.

A yogi is much more disciplined in his speech. Yogic tradition has it that speech must pass before three barriers prior to being uttered aloud. These barriers come in the form of three questions: Is it kind? Is it true? Is it necessary? If the idea pending expression can pass these three tests, it is worthy of being expressed. Otherwise the yogi should hold his tongue.

As we delve into this verse we can see that there is more than meets the eye. The seemingly whimsical example actually contains great insight into the transformation of superficial, sensory life into profound, spiritual life.

प्रकाश्यते क्वापि पात्रे ।

prakāśyate kvāpi pātre

prakāśyate—*is manifest*
kvāpi—*where there is*
pātre—*able vessel*

Verse 53:
Love is manifest where there is an able vessel.

This simple verse is one of the loveliest in the text. Narada states clearly that love is manifest where a capable vehicle is present; love abides where it is welcome. To the ordinary human personality, love is confused with obtaining one's desires and, as such, it appears as an elusive experience based on external acquisitions. To the ordinary spiritual aspirant, love is confused with obtaining some psychic or spiritual experience, such as a vision. Love then appears to be something that must be sought and, therefore, it remains an elusive experience based on externals.

The bhakti yogi, however, realizes that he is not seeking love, but that it is love that is seeking him. His task is not to make himself into something special, whereby he can acquire love; his task is to make himself into nothing, a vessel empty of selfish individuality. When the vessel is empty, then God can fill it with divine love. This emptying of the sense of egoic personality is referred to as "the great disappearing act." The ego disappears and love appears.

Nan-in, a Japanese Zen master during the Meiji era (1868–1912), received a university professor who came to inquire about Zen. Nan-in served tea. He poured his visitor's cup full, and then kept on pouring. Tea spilled onto the table and down on the floor.

The professor tried to remain dignified, but eventually he exclaimed, "The cup is full. Stop pouring, no more can go in!"

"Like this cup," Nan-in replied, "you are full of your own opinions and speculations. How can I show you Zen unless you first empty your cup?"

गुणरहितं कामनारहितं प्रतिक्षणवर्धमानम्
अविच्छिन्नं सूक्ष्मतरम् अनुभवरूपम् ।

guṇarahitaṃ kāmanārahitaṃ
pratikṣaṇavardhamānam avicchinnaṃ
sūkṣmataram anubhavarūpam

guṇarahitaṃ—*devoid of the modes of nature*
kāmanārahitaṃ—*devoid of desire*
pratikṣaṇa—*perpetual*
vardhamānam—*expanding*
avicchinnaṃ—*boundless*
sukṣmataram—*exquisitely subtle*
anubhavarūpam—*the form of intimate experience*

Verse 54:
This love takes the form of an intimate experience of exquisite subtlety—devoid of the influence of the three modes of nature, devoid of desire—a boundless, perpetual expansion.

Here Narada undertakes what he proclaimed in verse 51 was impossible: he attempts to express the love that is inexpressible.

This beautiful and stirring description of love speaks for itself and provides the aspirant with an inspiration to seek this grand state. The Vaishnavas in India describe this state as being one of ever-increasing bliss. Perhaps we aspirants can measure what we deem "happiness" in comparison to these descriptions, thereby avoiding settling for less than God holds for us as real happiness.

तत् प्राप्य तदेवावलोकयति, तदेव शृणोति, तदेव भाषयति, तदेव चिन्तयति ।

tat prāpya tadevāvalokayati tadeva śṛṇoti tadeva bhāṣayati tadeva cintayati

tat—*that [the experience of verse 54]*
prāpya—*achieving*
tadeva—*that only*
avalokayati—*sees*
tadeva—*that only*
śṛṇoti—*hears*
tadeva—*that alone*
bhāṣayati—*speaks of*
tadeva—*that alone*
cintayati—*thinks of*

Verse 55:
Achieving that experience one sees only love, hears only love, speaks only of love, and thinks of love alone.

To the one who experiences the state presented in the previous verse, the eyes, ears, mouth, and mind experience reality as an abundance of beauty and love. This is no poetic fancy! Just as the ordinary person sees the world through lenses of selfish desires, the love-infused yogi perceives reality as so many reflections of God.

I am fond of reminding my yoga students of the saying "It takes one to know one" when they become lost in condemnation and judgment of others. The world that we perceive is a reflection of our own states of mind and reveals our own level of consciousness. The world is little more than a Rorschach blot in which we see our own desire systems projected. We see what we want to see.

This is reminiscent of the humorous story about the man who went to a psychiatrist for consultation. The psychiatrist administered several Rorschach inkblot tests to evaluate his patient. For each inkblot the man described a scene filled with sexual activity. The psychiatrist raised the question, "Sir, don't you think it peculiar that you see sex in everything I show you?"

"What do you expect," replied the patient, "when all you show me are dirty pictures?"

Because the world we see is reflective of our own mind-states, change is actually possible. This change comes about through accepting responsibility for the world as we see it. Behavior is secondary; the crucial issue is that we do not blame God or others for our experience of the world. Our lives, our relationships, our consciousness have one master only—ourselves. No guru, nor God himself, would ever interfere with free will and impose his consciousness on us. We are fully responsible for our perception of the world and we are fully responsible for our spiritual progress.

An enlightened person is simply one who chooses to look

for God in all aspects of the worldly Rorschach blot. And by seeking, he will find. By choosing to see God, all petty, partial perceptions fall by the wayside, leaving the vision of God. Just as the patient saw the sex that he was looking for, likewise will the yogi see the God that he is seeking.

गौणी त्रिधा गुणभेदाद् आर्तादिभेदाद् वा ।

gauṇī tridhā guṇabhedād ārtādibhedād vā

gauṇī—*subordinate (here, "inferior spiritual devotion")*
tridhā—*threefold*
guṇabhedāt—*the various modes of nature*
ārtādibhedāt—*the various types of distress*
vā—*or*

Verse 56:
Inferior types of spiritual devotion are threefold: of the various modes of nature, or the various types of distress.

This verse and the next follow up a point made in verse 54 that love is *gunarahitam,* "devoid of the three gunas." The nature of the gunas was discussed in the commentary of verse 47, in which we examined how they form the three strands of the chord of bondage. The three types of inferior spiritual devotion referred to here are reflections of the three modes of nature and their respective three types of personal distress.

Common religious devotion is influenced by the three gunas. The majority of conservative religious traditions are responses to the needs of their members who are under the influence of these modes of nature. Those under the influence of tamas tend toward laziness and apathy, resulting in poor health, limited vigor, and general unhappiness. They are unable to perceive of religious life as anything other than relief of their pain. Their religious ideal becomes an idyllic state that can generally only be realized after the death of their burdensome physical body. This orientation is reflected in the various religious traditions that promise their followers heaven after death in exchange for belief in dogma during life.

Those individuals under the influence of rajas have a great deal of energy, but this energy tends to be hyperactive and dualistic. They see life as a battleground on which they must somehow fight and conquer evil influences on behalf of God. Their orientation toward religious life often takes the form of seeking great accomplishments, such as building large temples or converting masses of people to their chosen beliefs.

Those under the influence of sattva seek peace and serenity in familial and societal realms. They are often well intentioned, concerned with getting along with others and alleviating the pain of those who are suffering. They tend to experience God as a force of good, and they wrestle with different ideas about the nature of evil and how it can be overcome by peaceful good wishes. Those under the influence of sattva-based devotion are often found involved in social and political movements in which religion is called upon as a force to work in the world.

उत्तरस्मादुत्तरस्मात् पूर्वपूर्वा श्रेयाय भवति ।

uttarasmāduttarasmāt pūrvapūrvā śreyāya bhavati

uttarasmāduttarasmāt—*each one subsequent*
pūrvapūrvā—*each one previous*
śreyāya—*superior*
bhavati—*becomes*

Verse 57:
Each subsequent type of spiritual devotion is superior to the ones that preceded it.

This verse follows on the point made in the previous verse. Here Narada alludes to the superiority of each of the three levels of inferior devotion as compared to that which preceded it. Devotion under the influence of rajas is superior to that under the influence of tamas, and devotion under the influence of sattva is superior to both rajas- and tamas-influenced devotion. The emotional thrust of devotion under the influence of tamas is selfishness; under rajas it is passion; and under sattva it is compassion.

Deep bhakti surpasses these three levels of devotion because its emotional thrust is freedom. The great lovers of God leap from the edifice of social consensus and religious identity in order to soar in the sky of God's love. They have rendered unto God what belongs to God, and having found that everything belongs to God, they are unfettered in their minds and hearts. Being unfettered, they find the freedom for which all beings yearn. And being free, the soul spreads her wings and flies back into the heart of God.

अन्यस्मात् सौलभ्यं भक्तौ ।

anyasmāt saulabhyaṃ bhaktau

anyasmāt—*than others*
saulabhyaṃ—*easier*
bhaktau—*regarding devotion (here, "the path of spiritual devotion")*

Verse 58:
The path of spiritual devotion is easier than others.

This is the first of a set of three verses that relate to the nature of bhakti as a path of spiritual development. Here, in the initial verse, Narada states that devotion is *saulabhyam* (easier) than other spiritual paths. The reason that bhakti is easier is that the path of love, by its very nature, is one in essence with all spirituality. Love is the alpha and omega of all existence; it is the prime mover, originator, sustainer, and remover of obstacles. A spiritual path that is coordinated with love is bound to be easy since it is in harmony with the All that is God.

The nature of God is sat-chit-ananda—eternal truth, absolute consciousness, and the ever-increasing bliss of love. Sat (truth) and chit (consciousness) are also valid foci for aspiring yogis. As stated previously, jnana yogis aspire after sat and raja yogis aspire after chit. Relative to our experience as imperfect human beings, however, sat is remote and impersonal, and chit is static and difficult to approach.

The bhakti yogi seeks to know God through his ananda aspect, through love. The nature of love is that it yearns to include that which seems to lie outside of its scope, so the ananda aspect of God is both intimate and approachable.

The ananda aspect of God is that which descends to lift humanity, the grace discussed in verses 38–42. The bhakti yogi need not struggle to climb immense peaks of spiritual accomplishment; he need only raise his arms in true longing and he will be lifted to the very heights of love.

Many yogis experience spiritual life as a struggle against great forces that must be overcome through a process taking many lifetimes, with the possibility of failure always present. The bhakti yogi, however, learns to offer himself in simple humility before God, knowing how little his mind can know, how weak his efforts are, and how impotent his struggles in the face of the immensity that God's will accomplishes in the twinkling of an eye.

In this spirit, the bhakti yogi becomes an empty vessel in which God can pour his grace. The bhakti yogi finds that all aspects of spiritual life are accomplished because love is God's will. As Sri Ramakrishna said, "Bhakti, love of God, is the essence of all spiritual discipline. Through love one acquires renunciation and discrimination easily."*

Let us conclude this verse with the inspired words of Kabir:

O Sadhu! the simple union is the best.
Since the day when I met with my Lord,
there had been no end to the sport of our love.
I shut not my eyes, I close not my ears,
I do not mortify my body;
I see him with eyes open and smile, and
behold his beauty everywhere;
I utter His name, and whatever I see,

---

*Ram Dass, *Be Here Now* (New York: Hanuman Foundation, Crown Publishing, 1978), 75.

it reminds me of Him; whatever I do, it
becomes His worship.
The rising and setting are one to
me; all contradictions are solved.
Wherever I go, I move round Him,
All I achieve is His service:
When I lie down, I lie prostrate at His feet. . . .
I am immersed in that one great bliss which
*transcends all pleasure and pain.**

प्रमाणान्तरस्यानपेक्षत्वात् स्वयं प्रमाणत्वात् ।

pramāṇāntarasyānapekṣatvāt svayaṃ pramāṇatvāt

pramāṇāntarasya—*of any other proof*
anapekṣatvāt—*without necessity*
svayaṃ—*of itself (here, "self-evident")*
pramāṇatvāt—*being the proof*

Verse 59:
The proof of this is self-evident, needing no other proof.

Many spiritual traditions, both Eastern and Western, are concerned with philosophic questions of epistemology, the study of how what can be known comes to be known. The yogic tradition is no exception, and different schools provide different standards by which knowledge is considered valid.

*Kabir, *Songs of Kabir,* trans. Rabindranath Tagore (York Beach, Me.: Samuel Weiser, 1977), 89.

Patanjali, for example, cites three types of valid knowledge: accurate perception, logical inference, and authoritative testimony.

In this verse, Narada offers self-evident experience as a legitimate source of valid knowledge concerning bhakti. He refers to the power of direct experience that need not rely upon any external source of support. The one who touches upon devotion to God needs no logical support nor corroborative testimony. He simply smiles, knowing that he knows.

शान्तिरुपात् परमानन्दरुपाच्च ।

śāntirūpāt paramānandarūpācca

śāntirūpāt—*the nature of peace*
paramānandarūpāt—*the nature of supreme joy*
ca—*and*

Verse 60:
It is of the nature of peace and supreme joy.

This verse offers a succinct statement about the nature of the path of spiritual devotion. Peace and supreme joy may seem like end-states to practitioners on more difficult spiritual paths, but the path of devotion should be filled with peace and joy from the very beginning. Their absence is an indication that something is amiss.

I have met many spiritual aspirants over the years who seem to take pride in the difficulty of their spiritual practices and the apparent lack of progress they have made, even after many years of diligent sadhana. Carrying their weariness like battle scars, they congratulate themselves on the difficult and challenging venture they believe they are undertaking. They develop strong determination and willpower, maybe even siddhis, but peace and joy elude them.

This is not to give the false impression that the path of bhakti yoga is not demanding. But its demands are of a different nature. In bhakti, an aspirant must seek to see God face to face and resist any interferences that may arise. The primary interferences are the false thoughts that his ego will propose, tempting him to believe that God is not available to him here and now.

The ego attempts to convince the soul that she is, indeed, separate from God and must undergo some variety of transformation or growth in order to regain the unified state. The revelatory experience, however, has nothing to do with growth; it is transcendent. The eternal relationship of the soul and God must be present now. Eternal, after all, means eternal. Eternal does not mean a long period of time; it means that what has existence (sat) is present here and now, always. The ego offers as proof of the separative "reality" the evidence of the senses and the testimony of the rambling mind under the influence of rajas and tamas.

As the soul awakens to her actual identity, the influence of rajas and tamas wanes, and the mind becomes peaceful in the sattvic state. As the soul awakens to her relationship with God, she touches upon the ananda aspect of God—love and joy. On the bhakti path, the path and the goal are one and the same. Peace and joy serve, from the beginning of the path until its summation, as polestars of spiritual direction.

लोकहानौ चिन्ता न कार्या
निवेदितात्मलोकवेदत्वात् ।

lokahānau cintā na kāryā
niveditātmalokavedatvāt

lokahānau—*worldly losses*
cintā—*anxiety*
na—*not*
kāryā—*duty*
niveditātma—*dedication of oneself*
lokavedatvāt—*of worldly and traditional social duties*

Verse 61:
When one dedicates oneself to the performance of worldly and traditional social activities from a sense of duty, there is no anxiety about worldly losses.

Here is the first of a series of six verses that review the topic of how the bhakti yogi should relate to the world and social responsibilities. This topic was touched upon in verses 8 and 11, in which Narada recommended that the aspirant not deny participation in social duties. In this set of verses we have a more detailed examination of the state of mind of the yogi who is "in the world but not of it."

For most people, activities are performed or avoided based on egoic concerns with rewards and punishments. The great mass of people lead conditioned lives founded on performing "good" deeds in order to receive positive reinforcement—such as wealth, fame, or comfort—and not performing "bad" deeds in order to avoid consequences—such as poverty, infamy, or criminal prosecution. A life lived chasing after petty rewards and running away from punishments is a paltry existence. It is filled with worries and confusion, ever tenuous and unsure, built on social edifices that can never be counted on for sure footing.

Such a life can never satisfy one who has tasted of spiritual devotion. The deeds he performs arise from a sense of duty, that which he feels is proper based on his intuitive comprehension of God's guidance. The aspirant need not look in a law book to learn what is good or bad. He studies the scripture of his own heart, in which God has inscribed the simple rules that provide for all he needs to live a beauty dream of love and healing, and manifest a world without fear.

Because the yogi participates in, or refrains from, activities based on a sense of duty, he has no anxiety about their outcomes. He is not seeking positive reward or avoiding negative consequence. He finds satisfaction in a task itself. This is similar to those tasks that ordinary people undertake for pleasure and relaxation, such as vacationing and hobbies. To the yogi, life itself is a vacation and the tasks he undertakes are his hobbies. Mahatma Gandhi described his tireless service to the people of India as his delight and recreation.

Because he is the consummate artist, the yogi seeks beauty, harmony, and perfection in the performance of his tasks. Unlike most worldly artists, however, he is not driven by some angst to express himself through a particular medium. The yogi may choose to utilize a traditional art form as a medium, but he is just as likely to express himself artistically through common daily activities, such as eating, bathing, or driving to work. The mundane mind finds these tasks mundane, while the mind inspired by devotion finds them inspiring. The artful consciousness of the yogi arises from his sense of God's abundance, and this abundance spills out into his lifestyle like the nectar from a cup that runneth over.

न तत् सिद्धौ लोकव्यवहारो हेयः किंतु
फलत्यागः तत्साधनं च कार्यमेव ।

na tat siddhau lokavyavahāro heyaḥ kiṃtu
phalatyāgaḥ tatsādhanaṃ ca kāryameva

na—*not*
tat—*that [anxiety-free state of verse 61]*
siddhau—*perfection of*
lokavyavahārah—*interactions with the world*
heyaḥ—*forsaken*
kiṃtu—*rather*
phalatyāgaḥ—*relinquishment of fruit [of actions]*
tat—*that*
sādhanam—*means of development*
ca—*and*
kāryam—*duties*
eva—*indeed*

Verse 62:
A lack of perfection of that anxiety-free state does not imply that interactions with the world are to be forsaken; rather, duties should indeed be performed as a means of developing that state, by relinquishing their fruits.

This verse is reinforcement of the view that the aspirant is not to renounce worldly activities. Here Narada tells the aspirant not to use imperfection as an excuse to avoid performing actions in the world. Even if one has not fully attained the anxiety-free state referred to in the previous verse, he is still to act in the world. The world is not to be renounced or forsaken; it is to be transformed through devotion and loving service. Furthermore, duties are to be utilized as a means of developing that perfected state; performing proper actions becomes a form of sadhana.

Phalatyāgah [phalatyagaha], "relinquishing fruits of action," reflects the attitude of one practicing karma yoga (verse 48). He is engaged in his appointed duties without concern for results. He acts out of the compassion for suffering beings that arises spontaneously from his heart. The Tibetan Buddhists remark on the complementary phenomenon of compassion arising in one who realizes the insubstantiality of all form. Similarly, the bhakti yogi finds love for others spontaneously arising in his heart as a result of his dispassion toward the world.

The worldly person is intent on "getting" from the world; as such, he is continuously frustrated because there is always more to get. The yogi is intent on giving to the world; he enjoys contentment as there is always more to give. Even if his love and devotion are not perfect, he still remains active in the world, among his brothers and sisters, humbly serving God's children.

स्त्रीधननास्तिकचरित्रं न श्रवणीयम् ।

strīdhananāstikacaritraṃ na śravaṇīyam

strī—*women (here, "sex")*
dhana—*wealth*
nāstikaṃ—*nonbelievers (here, "worldly people")*
caritraṃ—*stories*
na—*not*
śravaṇīyam—*listen to*

Verse 63:
Stories about sex, wealth, and worldly people should not be listened to.

Even though the yogi is in the world, he is not to sleep in its muck. He is not to indulge in the meaningless games played by egoistic personalities. Narada here refers to three preoccupations of worldly people—sex, wealth, and gossip. The aspirant is to avoid becoming concerned with matters related to lust, wealth, and worldly accomplishments because these aspects of life are certain to distract him from his goal of cultivating supreme love.

What passes for communication in the world is often just idle chatter about matters pertaining to meaningless sex, ill-gotten money, or superficial people who have achieved fame. The yogi will eventually have enough personal power that, if he finds himself in an environment where these are the primary topics of discussion, he will be able to steer the conversation in a more conscious direction.

अभिमानदम्भादिकं त्याज्यम् ।

abhimānadambhādikaṃ tyājyam

abhimāna—*egoism*
dambha—*arrogance*
ādikam—*et cetera [and other iniquities]*
tyājam—*are to be relinquished*

Verse 64:
Egoism, arrogance, and other iniquities are to be relinquished.

This verse is a companion to the previous verse. In verse 63, Narada cautioned the aspirant to avoid becoming enmeshed in disruptive externals. Here he warns the aspirant against being entangled in internal distractions: egoism, arrogance, and other iniquities.

Egoism is the state of ignorance in which the soul believes herself to be a body/mind complex, labeled "a bag of skin" by Zen teacher John Daido Loori.* The ego, being part of the mental apparatus (verse 48), has no life of its own. It only functions when the soul shines her light on the mind. Avidya is the state when the soul confuses her identity with the limited reflection presented by the egoic aspect of mind.

The ultimate arrogance of the ego is expressed in its belief that it exists as an entity separate from God. The ego claims a might it does not possess: it cannot create a separation where none exists. The wave does not have the power to separate itself from the ocean. Regardless of its foolish assertions, the

*I heard Sensei Loori use this expression at a retreat in Burlington, Vermont, in 1981.

wave's life, potency, and very existence are fully dependent on the ocean.

The ego is not "evil" for this performance; it is simply its nature to protect, preserve, and extend a sense of personal identity. In its rightful place, the ego serves to keep the body and personality healthy by establishing and protecting boundaries (such as destroying viruses that may attempt to "invade" the boundaries of the body). But the ego should act as servant, not master. When the ego becomes the leader of mental activity, then all other mental iniquities, such as kama, krodha, moha (verse 44) (desire, anger, delusion) arise from its arrogance.

तदर्पिताखिलाचारः सन् कामक्रोधाभिमानादिकं
तस्मिन्नेव करणीयम् ।

tadarpitākhilācāraḥ san
kāmakrodhābhimānādikaṃ tasminneva
karaṇīyam

tadarpitākhilācāraḥ—*that [duty] sanctifies all activities*
san—*being*
kāma—*selfish desire*
krodha—*anger*
abhimāna—*egoism*
ādikam—*et cetera (here, "and other iniquities")*
tasmin—*in that (here, "as a duty" [verse 62])*
eva—*only*
karaṇīyam—*performing*

Verse 65:
Performing actions only as a duty sanctifies all activities, even when selfish desire, anger, egoism, and other iniquities are present.

This is the fifth of the series of verses that examines the performance of actions in the world as a duty. Here Narada offers words of direction and solace to aspirants who are painfully aware of their shortcomings and wonder if their labors in the world are at all worthwhile or meaningful.

The bhakti yogi is aware that his sole task is to become a vessel for God's love. The purer his heart and mind, the more a channel he becomes for subtle spiritual energies emanating from higher planes. When his purity is contaminated by iniquities of egoism, the channels are blocked and the transmission of spiritual energy cannot take place.

When the aspirant becomes aware of the degree to which iniquities permeate his consciousness, he may become disheartened, thinking that his worldly tasks can never be sanctified, that they continue to enmesh him in karmic cycles and bring no relief to suffering humanity. Here Narada informs the aspirant that his motivation is enough to render his activities sanctified. The aspirant need not be perfect to perform service in the world; he need but be striving toward perfection. He need not desire only God; he need but desire to desire only God. He need not be pure to love God; he need but be working toward purity. It is the yogi's duty to do his best to be a clear channel for love. It is God's duty to see divine love somehow reach the world.

Several commentators interpret this verse to mean that the aspirant should direct his iniquities toward God. It is sometimes held that any strong emotion directed toward God is beneficial. As such, even anger toward God can be considered a form of bhakti, a sort of "enemy" yoga. In the Bhagavata-Purana, this is called the yoga of hatred, *samrambha yoga.*

From a practical point of view, an aspirant could benefit from adopting the attitude that his iniquities should be directed toward God because then he can realize how self-destructive are his negativities. He only harms himself when he relishes selfishness and attack, regardless of whom he blames as the cause or toward whom he directs the negative energy. Anger, for instance, can only rise due to the frustration of selfish desires, and it is first destructive to the consciousness of the holder even before he directs it out upon the world. As the Buddha said, directing anger at someone is like throwing a hot coal at them: the coal will first burn the hand of he who wishes to cast it.

त्रिरुपभङ्गपूर्वकं नित्यदास्यनित्यकान्ताभजनात्मकं प्रेम कार्यं प्रेमैव कार्यम् ।

trirūpabhaṅgapūrvakaṃ nityadāsyanityakāntābhajanātmakaṃ prema kāryaṃ premaiva kāryam

trirūpa—*three forms*
bhaṅga—*breaking (here, "going beyond")*
pūrvakam—*previously*
nitya—*eternal*
dāsya—*devoted servant*
nitya—*eternal*
kāntā—*loving wife*

bhajana—*worship*
ātmakaṃ—*the nature of (here, "naturally")*
prema—*love*
kāryam—*duties*
premaiva—*love only*
kāryam—*duties*

Verse 66:
Going beyond the three forms of spiritual devotion previously mentioned, one's only duty is to love. One's duty is to love. The aspirant naturally worships God, like an eternally loving wife or eternally devoted servant.

This is the conclusion of the series of six verses in which Narada discusses the nature of duty to the world for one who is developing devotion. The three forms of devotion to be gone beyond are the three forms of bhakti influenced by the three gunas (verses 56 and 57). The devotion described here is of an exalted level, transcendent to the three modes of nature, as first described in verse 54.

Within the current context regarding duty, this verse states that the duty of the accomplished yogi is to love alone. He is to see all tasks as forms in which he might be a vehicle for God's love to manifest. He becomes a marionette in the hands of the great puppeteer, playing his role wherever God places him.

St. Francis of Assisi prayed, "Lord, make me an instrument of thy will." When the yogi begins to perceive clear guidance as to what this will expects of him, all conflicts are resolved. For all activities are potential vehicles for the expression of love. No task is too great or too trivial, for all are opportunities to manifest God's light. What is essential is that the yogi bring love to life; the form that he uses for this purpose is of lesser significance.

भक्ता एकान्तिनो मुख्याः ।

bhaktā ekāntino mukhyāḥ

bhaktaḥ—*devotee*
ekāntinaḥ—*one-pointed*
mukhyāḥ—*foremost*

Verse 67:
Foremost amongst devotees are those who are one-pointed.

This verse marks the beginning of seven verses in which the nature of high yogis is the theme. This idea, initially touched upon in verses 20–22, will be developed here. Narada makes the simple point that those bhakti yogis who are most advanced on the path of devotion are *ekāntinaḥ [ekantinaha],* "one-pointed." This one-pointedness is necessary if the aspirant is to attain the high degree of emotional preoccupation necessary to realize God on the devotional path.

One-pointedness is mandatory if one is to rise to the summits of achievement in any spiritual system. In raja yoga, one-pointedness results in the achievement of *samprajnata samadhi,* the state of "samadhi with cognition," a high level of meditative absorption. In the tantric traditions, one-pointedness is necessary for the aspirant to raise the kundalini energy up the spine and pierce the various knots that block its ascent. In jnana yoga, a one-pointed resoluteness to shatter false mental states is needed for success. In bhakti yoga, as we shall see in the next verse, one-pointedness has more of an emotional slant. This is consistent with bhakti having as its orientation the ananda aspect of God.

कण्ठावरोधरोमाञ्चाश्रुभिः परस्परं लपमानाः
पावयन्ति कुलानि पृथिवीं च ।

kaṇṭhāvarodharomāñcāśrubhiḥ parasparaṃ
lapamānāḥ pāvayanti kulāni pṛthivīṃ ca

kaṇṭhāvarodha—*choking voice*
romāñca—*horripilation [hairs standing on end]*
aśrubhiḥ—*tearfully*
parasparaṃ—*with each other*
lapamānāḥ—*conversing*
pāvayanti—*purify*
kulāni—*communities*
pṛthivīṃ—*the earth*
ca—*and*

Verse 68:
Conversing with each other with voices choking,
hairs standing on end, and tears in their eyes,
they purify their communities and the earth.

This verse provides a picture of the emotional nature of highly developed bhakti yogis. The references given to hairs standing on end and tears in the eyes describe those overcome with deep emotion. Furthermore, the devotees are conversing with each other in choking voices; they are sharing their intoxication with each other in *satsang* (spiritual companionship). The implication is that devotees have accessed the heights of emotional experience, which they share together in community. There is to be no inhibition on the part of one who desires to experience spiritual devotion.

Emotions as experienced by bhakti yogis are different from emotions as we generally think of them. Mundane, personality-based emotions are the result of experiences based on the pairs of opposites. Mundane emotions arise within a spectrum bordered by the two poles of pain and pleasure. These emotions are triggered as the result of external stimuli over which the person has no full control. The emotional experiences of bhakti are transcendent to the pairs of opposites and the three gunas. States of devotion can be experienced regardless of pain or pleasure, fame or dishonor, or other dualisms because they are the result of inner receptiveness.

The bhakti yogi is a surfer on the waves of God's love. External stimuli, such as music or art, may trigger devotional states; but it is the purified nervous system of the yogi that transmits sensory data to the inner altar, at which feelings are offered to God and become transformed into spiritual states. Even when emotions are triggered by external stimuli, the yogi retains control of how they affect him, and he uses this control to come closer to God.

Narada states that these advanced yogis also purify their communities and the entire planet. Although we may be reluctant to accept this statement as literal, we should try to understand how yogis purify their environments. This verse is not a metaphor; those who carry God's energy with them are the purifying force in the world, counteracting the negative thought-forms that the contemporary mass of humanity produces.

In verse 50 Narada presented the idea that a highly developed yogi assists others through his union with all souls. Here Narada elaborates the point, stating that the influence of a yogi extends into social realms. The yogi purifies his community because he exerts a subtle influence on all with whom he comes into contact. Each person is touched by him in some way and, whether they realize it or not, they carry the benefit of his blessing with them. The blessing is magnified if it is consciously received, but its effect remains in place regardless of the awareness of the recipient. As those who have received the yogi's blessing carry out their affairs, they carry some amount of his spiritual energy with them, spreading it throughout their families and communities. A man who wears a fragrant flower on his collar spreads a perfume wherever he goes.

Because of the siddhis that the yogi develops, his blessing need not be delivered in person. The positive thought-vibrations that he emanates extend to any mind that is receptive. Like a superpowerful radio wave, the yogi's thought currents travel through vast spaces and are available for the "listening" of any who choose to "tune in." By serving as an amplifier on the earth plane for subtle energies from inner realms, the yogi does great service for the entire planet. He makes manifest energies that otherwise would be inaccessible.

तीर्थीकुर्वन्ति तीर्थानि सुकर्मीकुर्वन्ति कर्माणि
सच्छास्त्रीकुर्वन्ति शास्त्राणि ।

tīrthīkurvanti tīrthāni sukarmīkurvanti karmāṇi sacchāstrīkurvanti śāstrāṇi

tīrthīkurvanti—*make holy*
tīrthāni—*sacred sites*
sukarmīkurvanti—*render beneficent*
karmāṇi—*deeds*
sacchāstrīkurvanti—*basis of authority*
śāstrāṇi—*sacred scriptures*

Verse 69:
Their holiness establishes sacred sites, they render actions beneficent, and their authority is the basis of sacred scripture.

God and the Devil were walking together one day. God leaned over and picked up a beautiful, radiant gem.

"What is that?" asked the Devil.

"This," said God, "is Truth."

"Give it to me," the Devil responded. "I'll organize it for you."

Every organized religion attempts to ritualize and codify spiritual reality. Religious institutions establish certain places, behaviors, writings, and persons as representative of God. This is not malevolent in itself; it is a perfectly suitable security blanket for the immature. But problems inevitably arise as the dogma of one religion conflicts with that of another. Thus are various holy wars, crusades, inquisitions, and other evils undertaken in the name of God throughout the ages.

There is no spirituality without the great souls. They are

the ones who carry the torch of spiritual consciousness. Places of pilgrimage, scriptures, rites and rituals, and all other religious paraphernalia simply point to this level of consciousness. When these accoutrements become more significant than the attainment of God-consciousness, a religion loses its vitality and becomes, at best, a benevolent social institution or, at worst, a force for prejudice and cruelty. The consciousness of an enlightened being is the basis for holiness in the human realm.

तन्मयाः ।

tanmayāḥ

tat—*that [those bhaktas]*
mayāḥ—*fullness [of God]*

Verse 70:
To them is the fullness of God.

During the heyday of Buddhism in China, many women became enlightened. Unfortunately the social structure of the society was such that these women could not take their rightful place as spiritual teachers. Many of them have become known as "tea ladies." During that time there were pilgrimage routes on which the monks would travel, visiting various temples, monasteries, and teachers. Along the footpaths the tea ladies set up small stalls at which they served tea, food, and sometimes unexpected grace to the traveling pilgrims.

There are many stories describing incidents where monks stopped for refreshment at these tea stalls and arrogantly addressed the proprietess. After some exchange the tea lady would subtly introduce a profound exchange that, if the monk was sensitive, would reveal the enlightened state of the woman before him. Stories relate how some monks were brought to enlightenment by these humble, nameless bodhisattvas.

To those such as the tea ladies of China is the fullness of God. History is unlikely to record their names and they are equally unlikely to be recognized and appreciated during their own time. But the pearl of great price belongs to them and there is nothing in the world that could provide more. They have gained their own soul, so they care not if they lose the whole world. The wise aspirant is not fooled by status or rank. He remains alert and receptive to teachers who may appear before him in costumes unrecognizable to those blinded by worldly superficialities.

मोदन्ते पितरो नृत्यन्ति देवताः सनाथा चेयं भूर्भवति

modante pitaro nṛtyanti devatāḥ sanāthā ceyaṃ bhūrbhavati

modante—*rejoice*
pitaraḥ—*forefathers (here, "ancestors")*
nṛtyanti—*dance*
devatāḥ—*shining ones [divine beings]*
sanāthā—*endowed with a master*
ca—*and*
iyam—*this*
bhūḥ—*the earthly sphere (here, "the world")*
bhavati—*becomes*

Verse 71:
Their ancestors rejoice, divine beings dance, and the world becomes endowed with a master.

The realization of those who have come to the fullness of God benefits all sentient beings in three ways. First, the ancestral line of a devotee reaches its climax with his consciousness. Like a tree that is cultivated over millennia, the force of biological evolution reaches its conclusion; the family tree bears its fruit in the form of the devotee.

Second, the *devas,* the shining beings of the astral realms ("angels," as they are called in the Judeo-Christian tradition), serve the evolving ego throughout the course of his entire evolutionary sojourn. Their work comes to conclusion as the ego finally reaches the maturity of soul-realization. The devas experience great joy and satisfaction when they observe the culmination of their efforts on behalf of the divine will. The celebrations of the devas at these times are like cosmic birthday parties, complete with celestial music and merriment.

Third, the earthly sphere has contributed the physical materials needed by the ego to experience, and finally to become liberated from, bondage. Like a mother, the world has provided for the struggling aspirant, often disciplining through the law of karma. Still, the consciousness of nature is in harmony with God's benevolence and, like a proud mother, she feels blessed when one of her "offspring" becomes enlightened.

नास्ति तेषु जातिविद्यारूपकुलधनक्रियादिभेदः ।

nāsti teṣu jātividyārūpakuladhanakriyādibhedaḥ

na—*not* } *(here, "irrelevant")*
asti—*there is* }
teṣu—*among them*
jāti—*birth (here, "ancestry")*
vidyā—*knowledge (here, "intellect")*
rūpa—*form (here, "appearance")*
kula—*family (here, "class")*
dhana—*wealth*
kriyā—*activity (here, "occupation")*
ādi—*et cetera [other social realities]*
bhedaḥ—*distinctions*

Verse 72:
Among them, distinctions of ancestry, intellect, appearance, class, wealth, occupation, and other social realities are irrelevant.

Among bhakti yogis there is no prejudice. Ideas of separation, judgment, and hatred known by mundane thinkers are absent from the minds of the foremost devotees. There is no racism, no sexism, no bigotry, intolerance, or partiality. Worldly status means nothing. Everyone is welcome to join the circle of devotional love; the more who join, the richer becomes the circle. The radiance of the heart leads the bhakti yogi to others of his kind, and together they shine out into the world like a beacon, calling all who feel separated in darkness to join the circle of love.

यतस्तदीयाः ।

yatastadīyāḥ

yataḥ—*since*
tadīyāḥ—*belong to him [God]*

Verse 73:
Since they belong to God.

This is the conclusion of the series of verses, beginning with verse 67, that discusses foremost devotees. Continuing the theme of the previous verse, Narada states that the reason no intolerance is felt by devotees is that they identify themselves with their true reality, as children of God. The worldly person, on the other hand, aligns himself with some physical or social identity and comes to believe that that is his reality.

The ego, by its very nature, is a competitive beast. It thrives on separation and is constantly comparing itself with others. It is proud before those whom it judges as having less, and it is jealous of those whom it judges as having more. The ego is intent on oppressing those who have less, because it senses they are jealous toward it. It is fearful those whom it deems inferior will revolt and somehow take away that which it feels makes it superior. Oppression is one primary means by which the ego maintains itself.

Similarly, the ego is intent on wresting away from those it deems superior the resources or qualities that it feels it lacks. As it recognizes that overt aggression might result in its being oppressed (aware that it will be treated as it intends to treat others), it is often passive-aggressive, using the camouflage of flattery and other social tricks to seduce the more powerful prey into surrendering what it seeks. Jealousy and aggression are additional means by which the ego maintains itself.

Ultimately, in its arrogance, the ego compares itself to God and, finding itself lacking, seeks to wrest from God what he has that the ego lacks—the position as creator of life. This psychological dynamic of ego intolerance and competition is the force behind the creation of the various myths of Lucifer, the fallen angel, who was kicked out of heaven by God for desiring to be ruler of hell rather than servant in heaven. We can understand that these myths are not ontological realities but projections of an internal, psychological process that takes place within the ego of a human being. When a person indulges in oppression, jealousy, or aggression, he is stationing himself in the mind-state of Lucifer. When he rids himself of these negative thoughts, he attains his divine, godly state, and the heaven of his consciousness remains free of these unwanted rebels.

वादो नावलम्ब्यः ।

vādo nāvalambyaḥ

vādaḥ—*speech (here, "intellectual explanations")*

na—*not*

avalambyaḥ—*a source of reliance*

Verse 74:

Intellectual explanations should not be relied upon.

It may be said that the spiritual journey is a pilgrimage starting in the mind and leading to the heart. That is, the aspirant must learn to still the ramblings of the dualistic mind in order to intuitively penetrate into the unitary source of consciousness, known in yoga as the *hridayam,* or "spiritual heart." This heart is not the center of mundane emotional states; it is the very root of consciousness. Awareness of God involves a shift from conceptual mental perceptions to direct spiritual vision.

The resolution of the problem of suffering is not to be found in thought. Theories and concepts are of no avail; only realization of one's true identity can resolve the pain of egoic illusion. No matter how much a man knows about the qualities of fire, no matter how proficient he is at lecturing others about the utility of heat, unless he strikes a match and feels the flames himself he will remain cold.

The great sage Ramana Maharshi has said, "All metaphysical discussion is profitless unless it causes us to seek within the Self for the true reality. All controversies about creation, the nature of the universe, evolution, the purpose of God, etc., are useless. They are not conducive to our true happiness. People try to find out about things which are outside of them before they try to find out 'Who am I?' Only by the latter means can happiness be gained."*

---

*Ramana Maharshi, *Be As You Are: The Teachings of Ramana Maharshi,* ed. David Godman (Middlesex, England: Arkana, 1985), 179.

बाहुल्यावकाशत्वादनियतत्वाच्च ।

bāhulyāvakāśatvādaniyatatvācca

bāhulya—*extensive* } *(here, "endlessly")*
avakāśatvāt—*space* }
aniyatatvāt—*uncertain*
ca—*and*

Verse 75:
They can go on endlessly without providing certainty.

If not so sad in its results, the phenomenon of aspirants trying to figure out that reality which is *beyond* the mind by using the tools *of* the mind would be funny. The ego constantly attempts to analyze, define, and conceptualize experience. If an aspirant wishes to give himself a headache and ulcer, he should attempt to reach that which transcends egoic experience while utilizing the techniques of the ego.

Spiritual reality is not irrational, but it is transrational. The highest thought capable by the rational mind is that there exists something greater than itself. But what is beyond its reach it can never grasp. The finite mind cannot know the infinite, because there lies the peace that surpasses its understanding. Those who know God have found him beyond the limits of the mind, and they know him with a certainty that theoretical understanding can never provide.

भक्तिशास्त्राणि मननीयानि तद्बोधकर्माणि करणीयानि ।

Bhaktiśāstrāṇi mananīyāni tadbodhakarmāṇi karaṇīyāni

bhakti—*spiritual devotion*
śāstrāṇi—*sacred scriptures*
mananīyāni—*reflected upon*
tat—*that [spiritual devotion]*
udbodha—*awakening*
karmāṇi—*actions (here, "practices mentioned in the scriptures")*
karaṇīyāni—*performed*

Verse 76:
Devotional scriptures should be reflected upon and the practices therein should be performed, as they awaken devotion.

The placement of this verse is notable in that it follows two verses that state that learning from theoretical materials is not conducive to the goal of the aspiring yogi. He needs experience, not ideology. In this verse, however, contemplation on devotional texts and the practices therein are recommended. The reason for this apparent change of direction is found in the use of the verb *mananīyāni [mananiyani]*, "reflected upon." The teachings in devotional scriptures are to be taken into the mind and allowed to sit there until they are absorbed and integrated. Food is eaten and digested in the stomach so that its energy can spread through the rest of the body. Likewise, the teachings of spiritual devotion are brought into the consciousness through reading; then, if properly "digested," the energy contained within can be spread throughout the entire consciousness of the aspirant.

I studied formally with a dharma heir of Roshi Phillip Kapleau. I was told that the roshi was fond of saying that the purpose of spiritual reading was to inspire the student to spiritual practice. Once reading had provided that inspiration, it had accomplished its purpose.

Spiritual literature can be a great aid to an aspirant, or it can be a terrible hindrance. If it is used to inspire practice, motivate compassion, and nourish devotion, it serves a very valuable purpose. If scriptural study is used for mere intellectual understanding, for pride of accomplishment, or as a substitute for actual practice, then one is taking in too much mental food, which is sure to result in intellectual indigestion.

सुखदुःखेच्छालाभादि त्यक्ते काले प्रतीक्षमाणे क्षणार्धमपि व्यर्थं न नेयम् ।

sukhaduḥkhecchālābhādi tyakte kāle pratīkṣamāṇe kṣaṇārdhamapi vyarthaṃ na neyam

sukha—*happiness*
duḥkha—*sadness*
icchā—*will (here, "selfish will")*
lābha—*obtain (here, "worldly gain")*
ādi—*et cetera [other personal concerns]*
tyakte—*relinquishing*
kāle—*time*
pratīkṣamāṇe—*at every moment enthusiastic*

kṣaṇārdham—*half an instant*
api—*even*
vyartham—*uselessly*
na—*not*
neyam—*should be passed*

Verse 77:
Relinquishing happiness, sadness, selfish will, worldly gain, and other personal concerns, at every moment enthusiastic, not even half an instant should pass uselessly.

This verse and the following provide a specific outline of those behaviors and attitudes that are to be renounced and those that are to be cultivated. Similar to Patanjali's list of five *yamas* and five *niyamas* (disciplines regarding actions toward ourselves and others), Narada provides the aspiring bhakti yogi with a list of six character traits to be relinquished and six to be cultivated. Let us briefly review the six traits cited in this verse that are to be relinquished.

1 and 2: Happiness and sadness. Happiness and sadness are the two polls of egoic experience. As Freud pointed out, the selfish personality has only two drives: he strives to obtain what he wants, which he calls happiness or pleasure, and he avoids experiencing what he does not want, which he calls sadness or pain. To the yogi, all experience is seen as one, as a means to help him cultivate devotion. All experiences have equal meaning and value.

3: Selfish will. Selfish will is a mind-state based on duality. One experiences his consciousness in separation from others and from God, resulting in a false sense of conflict and contest. The egoic personality experiences his will as being in competition with others for those things that he believes bring him happiness. The ultimate competition seems to be with God, as he believes God may not provide him with the pleasures he desires, so he must fend for himself. Instead of being at peace with what he has, he feels he has to fight for what he wants.

4: Worldly gain. Objects of the world bring happiness to an individual because he does not realize what he is perceiving. He does not see the objective reality of an object because he has projected onto it his desires and attachments, either positive or negative. He perceives objects symbolically, giving them values they do not possess. All objects of the world are two-edged: they can be used by the worldly person to cause himself bondage, or they can be used by the yogi to reveal God's love.

5: Other personal concerns. To be concerned with specifics in the world is to confuse form and content. All objects and events in the world are given meaning and value by the perceiver. When the perceiver realizes that he inherently possesses the peace of God, he will no longer seek that peace which he mistakenly thought to be in the external world.

6: At every moment enthusiastic. One of the most striking characteristics of accomplished yogis is that they seem to be ever active, without any sense of strain. As their minds are focused on God, they are not distracted with petty worries and anxieties, leaving them able to follow the flow of God's energy in their lives. One of my teachers, Kenneth Wapnick, has founded a center to promulgate the teachings of the Christian mystical path based on *A Course in Miracles*. Ken states that all he has accomplished is simply the result of opening himself to the energy of Christ. He truly experiences himself as nothing more than an instrument, as a violin might be in the hands of a master musician.

अहिंसासत्यशौचदयास्तिक्यादिचारित्र्याणि परिपालनीयानि ।

ahiṃsāsatyaśaucadayāstikyādicāritryāṇi paripālanīyāni

ahiṃsā—*nonviolence*
satya—*truthfulness*
śauca—*purity*
dayā—*compassion*
astikyādi—*faith in spiritual teachings*
cāritryāṇi—*personal integrity*
paripālanīyāni—*cultivating*

Verse 78:
Nonviolence, truthfulness, purity, compassion, faith in spiritual teachings, and personal integrity are to be cultivated.

The six character traits that Narada states as worthy of being cultivated are as follows:

1: Nonviolence. Nonviolence is an attitude of benevolence toward all living things. Aspirants often misunderstand the teachings of nonviolence to mean that they should somehow become passive and nonintrusive when wrongdoings occur. This is not the case at all. Nonviolence is to be practiced by holding others compassionately in one's heart, and then acting in a manner most conducive to dharma in a given situation. This is why Krishna, the great avatar himself, taught Arjuna in the Bhagavad Gita that it was his duty, as a warrior, to engage in combat. A soldier or police officer who desists from conflict because he holds some dogmatic ideology is not practicing nonviolence, but avoidance. Neem Karoli Baba was fond of saying, "Do what you must do with another, just never put them out of your heart."

The wise yogi, if faced with a situation requiring confrontation, can usually find a means of avoiding actual physical contact, as the following parable relates.

> A vicious snake was terrorizing a small rural village. The snake lived near the village well, and whenever anyone approached for water, the snake would strike. A wandering yogi heard about this situation and spoke with the snake, demanding that he no longer attack.
>
> During his next trip through the village, the yogi found the snake beaten and badly injured. The snake told the yogi that the village boys had realized he would no longer strike, so they had taken him by his tail and smashed him upon the ground. The yogi shook his head in dismay that the snake would take his words to such an extreme, failing to trust his own nature as a snake. "It is true," said the yogi, "that I told you not to attack. But I didn't tell you not to hiss."

2: Truthfulness. Truthfulness is the means by which a yogi realizes his consciousness is one with others and thereby experiences communion with them. To tell a lie to another, either overtly or covertly, by commission or omission, is to create a boundary between two minds. Lies are the techniques by which the ego attempts to establish its apparent separation, for lying is a means of avoiding respecting and loving another.

The truth, truly, sets one free. The one who always tells the truth need not harbor in his mind any thoughts that he is not ready to share, for he honors those with whom he speaks, acknowledging that they deserve to be told the truth. Mahatma Gandhi called secrets a form of violence; he perceived how a lack of openness and honesty is a means of disrespecting and degrading others.

A practice I recommend to those who say they want an intimate relationship with their spouse or friends is something I heard Ram Dass refer to as "guts ball." In guts ball, the two parties sit facing one another and, while looking each other in the eyes, reveal all that is in their mind. Regardless of how benevolent, malevolent, embarrassing, or inappropriate, all thoughts are brought out into the open. Many people say they want community, but they are unwilling to do what is necessary to experience communion. Guts ball is a powerful upaya.

3: Purity. Purity is cleanliness and orderliness of the body and external environment, with everything found in its proper place. Purity requires a yogi to care for his body and his property. It is a characteristic especially apropos for our times, when too many disrespect nature.

Honoring nature means caring for the temple of our individual bodies, as well as for the temple of our collective body, the earth. The macrocosmic environment should be treated with respect; the yogi should treat the earth and its resources with gratitude and waste not. Likewise, his microcosmic environment should be treated properly. For the bhakti yogi living in the world, his body and clothing need not be plush, but they should be sattvic. Similarly, his dwelling place will reflect the lucidity of his mind; it will be simple, orderly, and comfortable. Alan Cohen tells his students that if they want to achieve clarity of mind they should begin by cleaning their bedrooms.

4: Compassion. Real compassion is the extension of love from a mind unclouded by illusion as to the nature of suffering. The yogi sees how suffering is self-created. He does not, therefore, rush in to fix problems in situations in which the parties involved will not accept the solution.

The ego can seldom be addressed directly, because its nature is denial of responsibility. It is often difficult for the sage to help others because his message of self-responsibility and identity in God is perceived as threatening. The persecution of many great saints is evidence of the reactionary nature of most human beings. Still, Narada tells the bhakti yogi that he must cultivate compassion for those who are suffering, and he implies that the yogi must be prepared to render loving service whenever it would be helpful.

5: Faith in spiritual teachings. It is easy to give lip service in praise of God when things are going well. But it is in times of trial and tribulation that spiritual teachings provide their greatest blessings. Unfortunately, it is at these times when many aspirants abandon faith and seek solace in social and mental support systems. It is when times are hard that aspirants are given the opportunity to leap beyond the ledges of the known on the wings of faith. A friend of mine is a Sufi teacher of the dances of universal peace. When diagnosed with cancer, she said she came to understand why sadhana is called spiritual "practice." She perceived her cancer as an event her practice had prepared her to shoulder without losing faith.

6: Personal integrity. Integrity is a characteristic of the person who is harmonized within himself. His mind is not split by various agendas and conflicting desire systems. The result is a person whose thoughts, words, and deeds are consistent. This is a state that cannot be faked or forced, but can be cultivated and brought along through diligent spiritual practice.

सर्वदा सर्वभावेन निश्चिन्तैः भगवानेव भजनीयः ।

sarvadā sarvabhāvena niścintaiḥ Bhagavāneva bhajanīyaḥ

sarvadā—*always*
sarvabhāvena—*in all ways*
niścintaiḥ—*free of anxiety*
Bhagavan—*God*
eva—*alone*
bhajanīyaḥ—*to be worshiped*

Verse 79:
Always, in all ways, worship God alone; be free of anxiety.

This brief but beautiful verse gives direct advice to the aspiring yogi. God alone is to be focused on; love alone is to be one's polestar, everywhere and at all times. In stillness and in movement, while in the depths of meditative absorption and in the midst of worldly life: Release fear and anxiety; be at peace.

There comes a point when I can only appeal to the reader to sincerely make an effort to realize the profundity of what Narada states. Give yourself to God and release all the misery, concern, depression, fear, and guilt that would keep him from your consciousness. Place no idols of anxiety on the altar of your heart. Give love to God that you may feel his love for you.

स कीर्त्यमानः शीघ्रमेवाविर्भवत्यनुभावयति भक्तान् ।

sa kīrtyamānaḥ
śīghramevāvirbhavatyanubhāvayati bhaktān

saḥ—*he (here, "God")*
kīrtyamānaḥ—*sincerely venerated*
śīghram—*swiftly*
eva—*indeed [for emphasis]*
āvirbhavati—*becomes manifest*
anubhāvayati—*aware of the existence*
bhaktān—*devotees*

Verse 80:
Through sincere veneration, God swiftly becomes manifest in the awareness of devotees.

As we approach the end of the text, we reach a simple summation of what has preceded. Through veneration of God, through sincere love and respect, God appears in the consciousness of the devotee.

This is no idle statement. God is a reality and thousands of great lovers throughout history, in every land, have testified to his reality. You, reader, aspirant, who desire to solve the mystery of creation, to find and eliminate the cause of pain, you who seek to live in love and joy and peace, this verse is intended for you. Have faith. Seek the God who is, at this moment, seeking to shine into your consciousness.

Call him Father, Mother, Brother, Friend—call him by any name or no name. Just call upon love. There is a longing for love in every person that will one day be satisfied. Go toward God. Release your egoic defenses; welcome and allow his love into your heart. He yearns to have you know him.

त्रिसत्यस्य भक्तिरेव गरीयसी भक्तिरेव गरीयसी ।

trisatyasya bhaktireva garīyasī bhaktireva garīyasī

trisatyasya—*in the threefold reality*
bhaktiḥ—*spiritual devotion*
eva—*alone*
garīyasī—*greatest significance*

Verse 81:
In all the threefold reality, spiritual devotion alone is of the greatest significance; it is spiritual devotion alone that is of the greatest significance.

The *threefold reality* refers to the three realms of existence—the physical, astral, and causal. What is important for our concern is not the precise nature of the various realms, but the underlying truth that can serve us everywhere. No matter where our karma may take us, no matter in what incarnation we find ourselves, no matter what may be taking place in our environment, spiritual devotion brings forth the love lying potentially in every space/time matrix.

It is by devotion that our vibrations become purified and uplifted. It is by devotion that we heal and are healed. It is by devotion that we bless those who share our current level of consciousness, and by which we proceed to higher and more subtle levels. It is love alone that provides the context in which God is real.

गुणमाहात्म्यासक्तिरुपासक्तिपूजासक्तिस्मरणासक्ति-
दास्यासक्तिसख्यासक्तिवात्सल्यासक्ति-
कान्तासक्तिात्मनिवेदनासक्तितन्मयतासक्ति-
परमविरहासक्तिरुपा एकधा
अपि एकादशधा भवति ।

guṇamāhātmyāsaktirūpāsaktipūjāsakti-
smaraṇāsaktidāsyāsaktisakhyāsakti-
vātsalyāsaktikāntāsaktiātmanivedanāsakti-
tanmayatāsaktiparamavirahāsaktirūpā
ekadhā api ekādaśadhā bhavati

guṇamāhātmyāsakti—*cherishing the glorious qualities*
rūpāsakti—*cherishing the form (here, "spiritual forms")*
pūjāsakti—*cherishing ritual worship*
smaraṇāsakti—*cherishing constant remembrance*
dāsyāsakti—*cherishing service*
sakhyāsakti—*cherishing as a dear friend*
vātsalyāsakti—*cherishing with parental affection*
kāntāsakti—*cherishing as a loving wife*
ātmanivedanāsakti—*cherishing knowledge of the Self*
tanmayatāsakti—*cherishing oneness with*
paramavirahāsakti—*cherishing the supreme separation*
rūpā—*form*
ekadhā—*singular*
api—*though*
ekādaśadhā—*of eleven*
bhavati—*becomes (here, "manifests")*

Verse 82:
Spiritual devotion is singular, though it manifests as eleven forms: cherishing the glorious qualities of God, cherishing the spiritual forms, cherishing ritual worship, cherishing constant remembrance, cherishing service, cherishing God as a dear friend, cherishing God with parental affection, cherishing God like a loving wife, cherishing knowledge of the Self, cherishing oneness with God, cherishing the supreme separation.

This verse describes the traditional eleven forms in which bhakti can be expressed. The yogi can relate to his Beloved in the form of a personal relationship—as a friend, a child, a spouse. He can cherish God in traditional religious performances—honoring saints, holy sites, and scriptures. He can hold God dear in the form of union—as his own Self, or in samadhi. All forms of God are equally suitable for love. Whichever form most inspires the yogi is the proper form. As has been previously stated, what is of value is the degree of devotion a practice can produce, not the particulars involved. Any relationship that increases love is acceptable on the bhakti path.

The last form of bhakti mentioned is cherishing the supreme separation. In many ways this is the pinnacle of love for God, because it requires complete surrender. The yogi must be willing to lay aside all of his opinions, judgments, desires, and values, even those he may think of as spiritual or righteous. He must submit himself to God and accept all aspects of life, from the most sublime to the most horrible.

In this form of bhakti, the yogi strives to taste the nectar of love even in the depths of separative consciousness. This entails a willingness to extend love even while burning in the fires of despair or freezing in the ice of loneliness. Such a one raises from his heart the greatest courage, compassion, and dedication. Such a one is so sweet and tender, loving all that could be deemed unlovable. Such a one is strong and wise, offering forgiveness to the selfish egos who apparently cause so much pain, suffering, and death. Such a one blesses all.

When one has a vision of the nightmare that is *samsara* (life based on separative consciousness), one sees, as did Buddha, the immensity of suffering. One perceives the vast spheres of the universe of illusion containing naught but endless pain, frustration, and struggle. He sees sentient beings caught in bonds of self-created sufferings, their lives filled with meaningless and futile ego contests. The world appears, as described by Shakespeare through Macbeth, as nothing more than "a tale told by an idiot, full of sound and fury, signifying nothing."* Tooth and claw seem to be the law; the bigger and meaner the rat, the more he achieves in the rat race.

Such a powerful and disturbing vision can test not only faith, but sanity. It is in this state that the sincere aspirant may seriously wrestle with the question of suicide. But this is the prelude, the dark hour, before the rising of the sun of great faith, of *para-bhakti,* "supreme spiritual devotion."

The light of this faith, in the midst of the darkness of cold night, is the triumph of the reality of God over the illusion of separation, of love over fear. This was the accomplishment of Buddha under the bodhi tree and of Christ on the cross. This is the accomplishment of all who sincerely tread the path of spiritual devotion. Those who can love, when no evidence or reason to do so can possibly be found, have come to the eternal fountain of amrita, the nectar of supreme love.

Listen to Hafiz, the ecstatic Sufi poet of the fourteenth century, calling us:

Come, join the courageous
Who have no choice
But to bet their entire world
That indeed,
Indeed, God is Real.

**Macbeth,* William Shakespeare. Act 5, scene 5. The full quote is: "Life's but a walking shadow, a poor player, /That struts and frets his hour upon the stage, /And then is heard no more. /It is a tale/Told by an idiot, full of sound and fury, /Signifying nothing."

He Spins and Whirls like a Golden Compass,
Beyond all that is Rational,
To show this dear world
That Everything,
Everything in Existence
*Does point to God.**

इत्येवं वदन्ति जनजल्पनिर्भयाः एकमताः
कुमार-व्यास-शुक-शाण्डिल्य-गर्ग-
विष्णु-कौण्डिन्य-शेषोद्धवारुणि-बलि-
हनुमद्-विभीषणादयो भक्त्याचार्याः ।

ityevaṃ vadanti janajalpanirbhayāḥ ekamatāḥ Kumāra-Vyāsa-Śuka-Śāṇḍilya-Garga-Viṣṇu-Kauṇḍinya-Śeṣa-Uddhava-Āruṇi-Bali-Hanuman-Vibhīṣaṇa ādayo bhaktyācāryāḥ

ityevaṃ—*in similar ways*
vadanti—*proclaim*
janajalpaḥ—*popular opinion*
nirbhayāḥ—*fearless*
ekamatāḥ—*unanimously*

*Hafiz, excerpt from "A Golden Compass" in *I Heard God Laughing—Renderings of Hafiz,* trans. Daniel Ladinsky (Walnut Creek, Calif.: Sufism Reoriented, 1996), 45, 47.

Kumāra Vyāsa Śuka Sāṇḍilya Garga Viṣṇu Kauṇḍinya Śeṣa Uddhava Āruṇi Bali Hanuman Vibhīṣaṇa	*great exemplars of spiritual devotion*

ādayo—*et cetera (here, "and others")*
bhaktyācāryāḥ—*great teachers of spiritual devotion*

Verse 83:
In similar ways Kumāra, Vyāsa, Śuka, Śāṇḍilya, Garga, Viṣṇu, Kauṇḍinya, Śeṣa, Uddhava, Āruṇi, Bali, Hanuman, Vibhīṣaṇa, and other great teachers of spiritual devotion unanimously proclaim, fearless of popular opinion.

Narada lists thirteen specific figures whom he recognizes as *acharyas,* "great teachers," of the bhakti path. These are our spiritual ancestors who have established devotion as a yogic path. The vibrations of their efforts on behalf of our world exist to this day, and the faithful aspirant knows that they can still be called upon for guidance and support. They are one with Christ in the statement "I am ever with you." They are, briefly:

1. Sanatkumara, the guru of Narada and a "mind-born" (verse 30) son of God;
2. Vyasa (verse 16), compiler of the Vedas and numerous other works. Some sources report he is a disciple of Narada;
3. Shuka, son and disciple of Vyasa, was the narrator of the devotional scripture Srimad Bhagavat-Purana;
4. Shandilya (verse 18), author of the Shandilya Bhakti Sutras;
5. Garga (verse 17), renowned astrologer and author of the Garga Samhita;
6. Vishnu, God in the form of the sustainer, appearing in his incarnations as Rama, Krishna, and others for the upliftment of humanity;
7. Kaundinya, son of Sandilya and a great bhakti yogi;
8. Shesha, the mythic thousand-headed serpent said to support the fourteen worlds. Patanjali is considered an incarnation of Shesha;
9. Uddhava, a beloved intimate of Krishna. Their dialogue is recorded in the Uddhava Gita;
10. Aruni, a great sage and son of a great sage;
11. Bali, originally a demon king, grew into a great bhakti yogi through his interaction with Vishnu;
12. Hanuman, considered an incarnation of Shiva, was the powerful monkey devotee of Rama as described in the Ramayana;
13. Vibishana, the brother of the evil Ravana (verse 42), the Ramayana describes how he experienced a change of heart and became both a great devotee of Rama and a righteous king.

य इदं नारदप्रोक्तं शिवानुशासनं विश्वसिति श्रद्धते स भक्तिमान् भवति सः प्रेष्ठं लभते सः प्रेष्ठं लभते इति ।

ya idaṃ Nāradaproktaṃ śivānuśāsanaṃ viśvasiti śraddhate sa bhaktimān bhavati saḥ preṣṭhaṃ labhate saḥ preṣṭhaṃ labhate iti

yaḥ—*whoso*
idaṃ—*this*
Nāradaproktaṃ—*decreed by Narada*
śivānuśāsanaṃ—*divinely auspicious teachings*
viśvasiti—*fully believes*
śraddhate—*with faith*
saḥ—*that one*
bhaktimān—*endowed with spiritual devotion*
bhavati—*becomes*
saḥ—*that one*
preṣṭham—*Dearest Beloved*
labhate—*obtains*
saḥ—*that one*
preṣṭham—*Dearest Beloved*
labhate—*obtains*
iti—*thus (here, "finis")*

Verse 84:
Whoso fully believes and has faith in these divinely auspicious teachings decreed by Narada becomes endowed with spiritual devotion. That one obtains the Dearest Beloved. That one obtains the Dearest Beloved. Finis.

As we come to the conclusion of Narada's glorious work, we hopefully find ourselves closer to the state he describes—infused with devotion, near our Beloved. Our tale, the tale of all souls: a raindrop of Shiva falling to earth and becoming jiva. She lands on a leaf, trickles through the forest, and eventually enters a brook. She flows with the brook into a river. The river merges with the sea, where she experiences the bliss of union with the other raindrops in their great destination.

But even this is not her final fulfillment, for the force of evaporation pulls her from the ocean and lifts her into the sky. There she makes her home in the clouds, resting at peace, until the overflowing ananda of Shiva brings her to earth again in a torrent of rain.

Thus does the wheel of love ever turn.

Let us close with the inspired poetry of the beautiful Papa Ramdas, one of this century's greatest bhakti yogis:

Perennial springs of Love are bubbling everywhere.
Continuous streams of Joy are flowering everywhere.
Unbroken waves of Light roll on everywhere.
The great Truth itself holds the feast everywhere. *

---

*Swami Ramdas, *At the Feet of God* (Kerala, India: Anandashram, 1986), 3.

Index of Select Sanskrit Terms

Word	Meaning	Sutra
abhimāna	egoism	27, 64, 65
ācāryāḥ	great teachers	34
ahiṃsā	nonviolence	78
amṛta	nectar of immortality	3, 4
ananyatā	single-hearted	9, 10
anūragaḥ	intense longing	16, 49
Āruṇi	Sage Aruni	83
astikyādi	faith in spiritual teachings	78
ātma	Self	6, 18, 66, 82
Bali	Sage Bali	83
Bhagavad	God	37, 38, 79
bhajana	worship	36, 66, 79
bhaktaḥ	devotee	67, 80
bhakti	spiritual devotion	1, 58, 76, 81, 84
bhaktyācāryāḥ	teachers of spiritual devotion	83
bhūḥ	the earthly sphere	71
Brahmakumāraḥ	son of Brahma (Narada)	30
buddhināśa	loss of buddhi	44
cāritryāṇi	personal integrity	78
dambha	arrogance	64
dāsya	servant	66, 82
dayā	compassion	78
dhana	wealth	63, 72
duḥkha	sadness	77
duḥsangaḥ	negative companionship	43
dveṣṭi	hate	5
ekāntinaḥ	one-pointed	67
Garga	Sage Garga	17, 83
grāhyā	worthy of being attained	33

Word	Meaning	Sutra
guṇa	attribute, mode of nature	37, 54, 56, 82
Hanuman	Hanuman	83
icchā	selfish will	77
Īśvarasya	of the Lord	27
jñāna	wisdom	6, 22, 25, 28
kāma	selfish desire	7, 44, 54, 65
karma	activity	25, 48, 69, 76
kāryā	duty	61, 62, 66
Kauṇḍinya	Sage Kaundinya	83
kīrtyamānaḥ	sincerely venerated	80
krodha	anger	44, 65
kṛpā	grace	38, 40
Kumāra	Sage Kumara	83
lokaḥ	of the world	8, 11, 14, 37, 47, 50, 61, 62
mahat	great souls	38, 39, 48
mattaḥ	spiritually intoxicated	6
mayāḥ	fullness	70
māyām	the [ocean] of Great Illusion	46
moha	delusion	44
mumukṣubhiḥ	those who aspire for liberation	33
Nārada	Sage Narada	19, 84
nirdvandvaḥ	free of the pairs of opposites	48
nirmamaḥ	without "I" sense (egoless)	46
nirodhaḥ	inner stillness	7, 8

Word	Meaning	Sutra
niścintaiḥ	free of anxiety	79
nistraiguṇyo	free of the three modes of nature	47
notsāhī	without passion for personal concerns	5
nyāsaḥ	consecration	8
parama	supreme	2, 19, 60, 82
Pārāśaryaḥ	son of Parasara (Sage Vyasa)	16
pātre	able vessel	53
phala	fruit	26, 30, 62
pramāṇa	proof	59
prema	love	2, 51, 66
preṣṭham	dearest beloved	84
pṛthivīm	the earth	68
pūjā	ritual worship	16, 82
rūpā	nature of, form	2, 26, 72, 82
sādhanam	means of development	28, 34, 62
sādhyatāṃ	cultivate	42
Śāṇḍilya	Sage Shandilya	18, 83
saṇgaḥ	companionship	35, 39, 45, 46
sannyasyati	renounces	48, 49
śāntirūpāt	the nature of peace	60
śāstra	scriptures	12, 69, 76
satya	truthfulness	78
Śeṣa	Shesha	83
siddhaḥ	perfect	4, 62
smṛtibhraṃśa	deprivation of memory	44
śraddhate	with faith	84

Word	Meaning	Sutra
śravaṇa	listening	37, 63
Śuka	Sage Shuka	83
sukha	happiness	24, 77
svarūpā	essence	3, 51
tīrthāni	sacred sites	69
tṛptaḥ	fully satisfied	4
tyāgaḥ	relinquish	10, 43, 46, 47, 48, 64, 77
udbodha	awakening	76
Uddhava	Sage Uddhava	83
vedān	the Vedas	49
vidyā	knowledge	72
vismṛti	forgetfulness	22
Viṣṇu	Lord Vishnu	83
viśvasiti	fully believes	84
viviktasthānaṃ	solitude	47
Vraja	Vrindavan	21
Vyāsa	Sage Vyasa	83
yogakṣemaṃ	concern for acquisitions which provide happiness	47
yogebhyaḥ	of traditional yoga	25

Bibliography

In preparing this book I consulted the following translations and commentaries of Narada's Bhakti Sutras. I would like to extend my respects to those who previously contemplated Narada's great work.

de Bary, Wm. Theodore. *Narada, Aphorisms on Devotion,* vol. 1 (Sources of Indian Tradition, n.d.)

Chinmayananda, Swami. *Narada Bhakti Sutra* (Bombay: Central Chinmaya Mission Trust, 1990).

Jyotir Maya Nanda, Swami. *The Yoga of Divine Love* (Miami: Yoga Research Foundation, 1982).

Prabhavananda, Swami. *Narada's Way of Divine Love* (Madras: Sri Ramakrishna Math, n.d.).

Shastri, Hari Prasad. *The Narada Sutras: The Philosophy of Love* (n.p., 1947).

Sinah, Nandlal, trans. *The Bhakti Sutras of Narada,* vol. 7 of *The Sacred Books of the Hindus* (New York: AMS Press, 1911.)

Sivananda, Swami. *Narada Bhakti Sutras* (Tehri-Garhwal, India: Divine Life Society, 1988).

Taimni, I. K. *Self-Realization Through Love* (Adyar, India: Theosophical Publishing, 1975).

Tyagisananda, Swami. *Narada Bhakti Sutras* (Madras: Sri Ramakrishna Math, 1955).

To contact the author write to:

Prem Prakash
Green Mountain Schoool of Yoga
40 Court St., Unit 3
Suite 216
Middlebury, Vermont 05753
USA

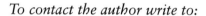